Clinical Knowledge and Practice in the Information Age:
a Handbook for Health Professionals

Jeremy C Wyatt DM FRCP

© 2001 Royal Society of Medicine Press Limited
1 Wimpole Street, London W1G 0AE, UK
207 Westminster Road, Lake Forest, IL 60045, USA
http://www.rsmpress.co.uk

British Library Cataloguing in Publication Data
A catalogue record for this book is available from the British Library

ISBN 1-85315-483-0

WX 216
IS IT
DEL HC
COMPUTERS

WX 26.5
MEDICINE
QUAL HC

Typeset by Dobbie Typesetting Limited, Tavistock, Devon
Printed in Great Britain by Bell & Bain Limited, Thornliebank, Glasgow

Contents

Foreword

The report *Health Care 2020*, launched in December 2000 as part of the Government's foresight programme, recommended the creation of a National Health Informatics Forum and identified as a crucial challenge the use in healthcare of 'innovative ways of exploiting knowledge and information to prevent disease and disability'. This requirement is of key importance, not only for industry, but for healthcare and the public sector more generally. The relevance of the efficient and imaginative use of knowledge to commercial competitiveness is clear, and, as shown by a study of European companies by Warwick Business School, one characteristic of successful firms is the investment in horizontal communications to encourage knowledge transfer.

In one sense medicine and the health sector have done well. There is a strong research culture and, in recent years, a growing commitment to the use of research results in decision making. The availability of a large pool of clinical trial outputs, for example, has permitted the Cochrane Collaboration to distil out reliable conclusions for practical use. The presence of a substantial if patchy evidence base has also made initiatives such as the National Institute of Clinical Excellence possible.

In another sense, however, the health sector's performance has been disappointing and fallen short of what might have been expected given the wealth of information that is potentially available to clinicians, managers and policy-makers. One problem has been the constraints imposed by healthcare organizations where computing and other relevant infrastructures are often deficient and where communication across institutions, and particularly across sectors of care, is generally weak. There are other shortfalls. For example, the vast body of routine information that is collected or that could be collected is insufficiently exploited, and there are large gaps in knowledge not only about treatment but also about diagnostic methods and the natural history of disease.

Despite this, the health sector should be is favourably placed to demonstrate how a large complex service could create a coherent system for producing, analysing, synthesizing and using knowledge to effect positive changes, to enhance performance and to make efficient use of human and financial resources. However, to date technological preoccupations have predominated and it is doubtful whether many major institutions—teaching hospitals for example—have either a well-conceived knowledge management strategy or the expertise to develop this type of activity.

Jeremy Wyatt is one of a small but growing number of clinicians who have seen the central place that knowledge management must take in future healthcare. It is timely that some of his experience in this field is now drawn together and made available through this publication. This collection of papers should provide a stimulus for senior managers, clinicians and policy-makers to consider how a knowledge management function might be incorporated into health services at all levels including hospitals, primary care and government departments.

Sir Michael Peckham
School of Public Policy, University College, London

Preface

'Our success depends on how well we exploit our most valuable assets: our knowledge, skills and creativity . . . the key to designing high-value goods and services . . . the heart of the modern, knowledge driven economy' [The Prime Minister, The Rt Hon Tony Blair MP, 1999].

Healthcare depends on huge amounts of knowledge derived from R & D and experience and applied by clinical 'knowledge workers'. However, despite the fact that three-quarters of healthcare costs depend on the knowledge-intensive decisions made by clinicians[1], health systems have invested little on managing this precious asset. In a recent study, 575 senior UK decision makers judged the public sector worst of the four studied on access to knowledge and working practices, lagging behind in organizational flexibility, customer focus and capacity for innovation[2]. This contrasts with equally knowledge-intensive sectors such as management consultancy and high tech industry, where knowledge management is already a £2 billion business and growing fast[3].

Knowledge management means recognizing the importance of knowledge and mobilizing it in a form that professionals can apply. Put this way, knowledge management has a long history, dating back to the invention of clay tablets 5000 years ago[4,5]. A wide range of technologies have developed since then (see Box).

Modern communications and information technologies, exemplified by the Internet, Intranets and decision support systems, thus need to be considered in the broader context of this range of tools and techniques which include paper 'systems' such as books and journals, hybrid systems such as bibliographic databases and person-to-person methods such as continuing education courses and secondments. The goal of this book is to help clinical professionals understand how to get the best out of these methods, to assist them with improving their own clinical knowledge and that of others (including patients and the public) and to participate in health service innovation, the core of initiatives such as the NHS Plan.

My thanks to Betsy Anagnostelis for her assistance with Chapter 4, Sir Michael Peckham for his continuing encouragement and provocative foreword and to Robin Fox for his careful editing of the 10 articles which first appeared in the *Journal of the Royal Society of Medicine* on which this book is based. I am also grateful to Justin Keen, Helen King, Henry Potts, David

Box Some key developments in the history of knowledge management

3000BC	Cuneiform writing on baked clay tablets — bulky and heavy
2800BC	Ink on papyrus — portable; libraries built
400BC	Socratic discourse and Aristotelian story telling
	Hippocrates demythologizes the 'sacred disease' (epilepsy), compares fertility of Scythian women with that of slave girl controls
200BC	Ink on parchment — expensive, but lasts for centuries
100AD	Ink on paper — cheap but fragile, susceptible to fire, one off
200AD	Galen's 83 treatises on medicine
700AD	Illuminated manuscripts produced by monks in scriptora
Ninth C	First medical school founded in Salerno
1200	Contents pages and indices appear — first information retrieval mechanisms
1300	Medieval guilds develop and formalize apprenticeship learning systems
1290	First case reports — Alderotti's Epistolae Medicales
1450	First printing press — books and leaflets become affordable
1522	Paracelsus attacks Classical dogma, lectures in German not Latin
1605	Bacon emphasizes observation as primary method of science, develops taxonomy of scientific knowledge, states 'Knowledge itself is power'
1664	First scientific journal, *Phil Trans R Soc Lond*
1670s	Sydenham writes up classic cases as disease portraits
1702	Peer review applied to J de Scavans
1761	Morgagni's 'de Sedibus', a disease encyclopaedia with causes and symptoms
1812	*N Engl J Med* founded
Nineteenth C	Growth of local libraries and information services
1880s	Dewey decimal classification for library catalogues
1930s	Atanasoff Berry computer, Colossus at Bletchley Park 1940
1940s	Human resources, continuing professional development activities
1949	Shannon formulates information theory
1954	Nash's 'Logoscope', a slide rule to assist diagnosis
1959	Hollingsworth: first computer aid (for diagnosis of lung cancer)
1966	Medline database launched
1973	Early medical 'expert' decision support system, MYCIN
1975	Clinical algorithms applied in Africa by Ben Essex
1980	Bernstein's electronic Hepatitis Knowledge Base
1985	Weed's Problem-Knowledge Coupler
1986	Oxford Database of Perinatal Trials, precursor of Cochrane Library — Chalmers
1992	Cochrane Collaboration founded; Web technology in use at CERN, Geneva
1995	World Wide Web takes off; first medical portals
1997	Intranets give staff access to internal and external knowledge sources
1999	Intelligent agents track Internet queries, suggest other resources of interest
2000	Over 200 free medical journals online; NHSDirect decision support system handles 16 million calls per annum; NHSDirect online provides public information

and Sylvia Wyatt for useful discussions and insights and to the BUPA Foundation for a 3-year programme grant which supported the UCL Knowledge Management Centre during the writing of the series and the book. As always, my family have been extremely patient during this process; without their support and encouragement it would never have happened.

JEREMY C WYATT

Director, Knowledge Management Centre,

School of Public Policy, University College London, UK

References

1   Tierney WM, Miller ME, Overhage JM, McDonald CJ. Physician order writing on microcomputer workstations. *JAMA* 1993; **269**: 379–83

2   Murray L. Releasing the value of knowledge: a survey of UK industry by Cranfield School of Management [www.microsoft.com/uk/knowledgereport]

3   Gordon D, Hamscher W, King D, Mueller A, Parker B, Retter T, eds. Knowledge management. In: *Technology Forecast*. Menlo Park, CA: Price Waterhouse Coopers Technology Center, 2000: 685–718

4   Goldberg A. Towards European medicine: an historical perspective. *J R Coll Physic Lond* 1989; **23**: 277–86

5   Newing R. From ancient Greeks to modern databases: In: *Knowledge Management Survey, Financial Times* business solution series, 28/4/99. London: Financial Times, 1999

1 Introduction: clinical questions and information needs

Experienced doctors differ from inexperienced doctors primarily in the amount and kind of knowledge they possess and their skills in applying it. In the commercial sector, professional knowledge is now seen as a rare and precious asset to be cherished, mobilized and communicated to improve the quality and efficiency of services[1]. This 'knowledge management' activity has a parallel in medicine—the evidence-based health movement, which focuses on managing evidence, a special form of knowledge[2]. However, despite worldwide uptake of evidence-based health, medicine still has a long way to go to match the care and resources spent on managing knowledge in other sectors. Doctors also need to debate as a profession whether and how to apply commercial knowledge management techniques in health.

One aim of this book is to contribute to that debate by summarizing what we understand about medical knowledge and how to manage it. It also has a very practical purpose—to help working clinicians improve their own knowledge management activities and those of their organizations, whether in keeping up with the published work or selecting, writing and using practice guidelines and computer packages (Figure 1.1). We start with clinical questions and how to deal with them.

Formulating clinical questions

All of us, from time to time, require further information to guide patient management—details of a drug side-effect, a test result, disease stage. The information may be needed to help an immediate decision about a patient, or less urgently to guide the future management of other patients or reorganize our clinical practice. The types of information needed and frequency of needing them were reviewed in 1996[3], and an important study of 1100 clinical questions posed by US family physicians was reported by Ely and others in 1999[4]. One key point that emerged was that the frequency of clinical questions varies according to context

1

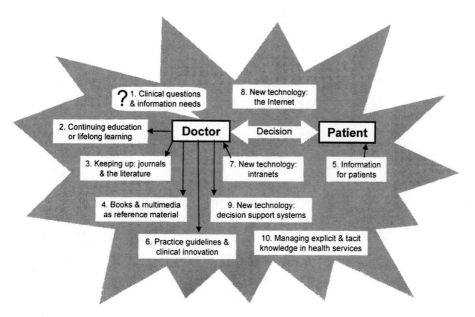

Figure 1.1 **Structure of 'Knowledge for the Clinician'**

and how a question is defined. An average is two clinical questions for every three patients[5]. The most frequent single topic about which information is sought is drug points[6]; in a primary-care study[4], at least one-fifth of questions concerned drugs.

The general rate of pursuing clinical questions was low—36% in a US primary-care study[4] and 12% in a UK inpatient study[7]. However, questions about drug dosing were pursued much more frequently, on 85% of occasions; perhaps doctors thought these were most likely to be answered satisfactorily. Overall, answers were found to 80% of the questions pursued.

Making the question clear

A clinical colleague calls you, asking you to tell her about aspirin and arthritis

It is hard to answer such requests for information without knowing the full context of the enquiry. How much detail is wanted? Will the information be used in patient care, or education, or research? And so on. Even knowing that the question is about patient care does not help much: is she uncertain about treating a rheumatoid patient with aspirin, about the risk of aspirin aggravating coexistent asthma, or about using daily aspirin consumption to measure pain intensity?

To generate a clear and useful answer to a colleague's question you need four specific kinds of information—the clinical dilemma (diagnosis, choice of tests, choice of therapy, etc.); the

Table 1.1 The elements of a well-formed question

Clinical dilemma	Possible clinical goals	Options being considered	Relevant patient data
Diagnosis	To select a test, select a therapy, identify a side-effect, give a prognosis, write a legal report . . .	Candidate diseases or complications of therapy . . .	Clinical and laboratory findings; past history and therapy
Choice of investigation	Disease staging, prognosis, monitoring therapy, patient reassurance . . .	No testing; list of tests and diseases to be distinguished . . .	Diagnosis, clinical findings, drugs; past test results; patient utilities and aversion to risk
Referral plan	Further investigation, access to restricted therapy, second opinion, social care . . .	No referral; to a peer in same institution; to another general hospital or tertiary centre; inpatient or outpatient . . .	Unexplained features, disease progression, previous therapy, patient dissatisfaction, social circumstances
Prognosis	To change or withdraw therapy, order further tests, counselling, reassurance . . .	Precise figure or rough prognosis (same, worse, or better than before)	Disease and stage, findings, test results; reason for patient's request for information
Choice of therapy	To prevent or cure; symptom control . . .	No treatment; names of treatment options; treatment regimens	Disease and stage; past therapies; allergies; patient tolerance of side-effects, risk, needles . . .
Follow-up schedule	Change of therapy, review of disease progress, review of test results, reassurance	No follow-up; where and how frequently to follow-up	Diagnosis; stage and stability of disease; patient self-care ability; duration of therapy; time till test results available . . .

clinical goal; the options being considered, including those already tried or dismissed; and patient data such as diagnosis, previous illness and current clinical findings. The specific information that needs to be communicated in the question varies according to the clinical dilemma; some examples are given in Table 1.1. This need for contextual information applies whether you are seeking the answer by asking a peer, searching the published work or even planning a research project. Table 1.1 places in this broader context the 'well-formed question' advocated by practitioners of evidence-based medicine[2]. Sometimes, if we formulate a clinical question in the way suggested and supply missing information (about clinical goals, the options being considered and relevant patient data), we can immediately perceive the answer for ourselves. More often, we will need to check with colleagues, books or other sources.

Answering clinical questions

You are visiting a patient at home and need to know the risk of aspirin aggravating asthma

Sometimes we can postpone seeking the answer till the consultation is over. We can look it up between patients or later, and write the answer in the notes. Often, however, the answer is critical to further action and cannot be postponed— and the patient probably knows it. The choice then lies between local print resources (books, journals, reprints), asking a colleague, and using a computer. Table 1.2 shows the commonest sources used by Ely's 103 family doctors to answer the 444 clinical questions they pursued, how long they spent seeking answers, and their success rates[4].

Wall posters were the fastest source and were usually helpful; but, probably because they can hold only a few pages-worth of information, they were seldom used. Calling a peer and looking up drug information in a book had high success rates and access times were acceptable at about 1 minute. Looking up other information in books or articles took 20 seconds longer than drug information and was less successful but was one of the most frequently used methods, presumably because books cover a very wide range of information. Finally, computers usually failed to provide the answer and took three times as long. This is probably why they were seldom used.

Instant clinical reference books

Factors that make a book suitable for instant reference include logical organization and indexing and judicious layout[8]. Familiarity also makes a big difference as it helps us to remember whether the information is there at all and where to find it. Obviously, the factual content of a clinical reference book should be as up to date and evidence-based as possible.

Table 1.2 Sources used by Ely's 103 family doctors to answer 444 questions, how long they spent seeking answers, and their success rate [Data from Ely *et al.* (Ref 4)]

Information source used	Per cent (No.) of questions pursued	Median time spent seeking answers	Success rate of searches
Peer: doctor, pharmacist, etc.	36% (161)	1 min 8 s	79%
Non-drug books, articles	32% (143)	1 min 10 s	52%
Drug texts	25% (113)	50 s	85%
Wall posters	4% (17)	35 s	82%
Computer databases, Internet, etc.	2% (10)	3 min	20%

When textbooks and review articles are written in the traditional way, several years can elapse before incorporation of clear evidence from primary studies[9]; thus, many authors and editors now conduct systematic literature searches to ensure that nothing important has been omitted. A good example is the *Clinical Evidence* series[10], which provides evidence-based answers to clinical questions. These answers depend on exhaustive literature searches updated every 6 months, with predefined methods for selecting, extracting and combining evidence[11]. A clinical reference book which still uses the informal approach but is well organized, comprehensively indexed and regularly updated is the *British National Formulary*.

Of course, books are of no value if they are out of date or missing from your shelf or library. The broader issues of selecting and maintaining a collection of books or multimedia are addressed in the next chapter.

Discussion with peers

Talking with a colleague often seems the best option when we are uncertain what to do, but a study of clinical communications in a Bristol hospital showed that many of the phone calls were unsuccessful attempts to locate the right person[12]; the moral is that organizations should improve their phone directories. Voicemail has perhaps made matters worse, but mobile phones should improve communication.

Even if we do succeed in making such contact, discussions of this sort have disadvantages: peers expect us to remember their answers, resent interruptions during cardiac bypass procedures or ward rounds, may expect favours in return and prefer not to be disturbed from 2200 h to 0800 (when many clinically important questions arise). Some peers are displeased when we do not take their advice or call someone else. Often we must compromise between talking to the most appropriate person and the most available person—the professor of neurosurgery, for instance, versus a colleague next door. A third alternative is to consult an information service that helps refine a question, search for the answer and return a summary within a few hours; several now exist around the UK (R Stamp, personal communication).

Studies of the behaviour of large communities of doctors[13] have shown that there is usually a small core of 'opinion leaders' who field most of the difficult clinical questions. These are often the clinicians who engage in teaching and research, travel to conferences and keep in touch with the published work. Such networks can be formalized by providing telephone help lines manned 24 hours a day[13]; however, since these same opinion leaders often sit on guidelines committees, one can also access their wisdom indirectly. Guidelines can be useful in answering routine clinical questions, but you may have difficulty in finding the ones you need[14], in resolving differences between them[15] and in checking which part refers to the current clinical dilemma. Guidelines are discussed in Chapter 6.

Instant access to computers

Table 1.2 shows that, regrettably, computers are not yet the ideal way to get satisfactory and speedy answers to clinical questions. Clinicians in Ely's study sought computer-based information in only 10 (2%) of the 444 questions they tackled[4]. Further evidence of low usage rates for electronic information resources comes from a systematic review[6] showing rates of between 0.3 and 6.7 per month for practising US doctors. It is noteworthy that doctors used Medline to answer two-thirds of their questions when electronic textbooks and full-text journals were also available[6]. Even with the help of an experienced librarian, Medline is helpful in only half of primary care dilemmas[16]; this suggests either that the doctors needed training in this respect or that their questions were often related to research rather than practice.

Thus, despite the predictions of Lawrence Weed, with his 'problem-knowledge coupling' software[17], and Sackett's pioneering work with a computer on teaching rounds[7], paper still seems to win hands down. Doctors should not be reluctant to use computers because of patient anxiety. Johnson *et al.* found that patients were more satisfied with a consultation if the doctor, when in doubt, used a computer rather than a book[18]. Doctors' reluctance to use computers may stem from difficulty in finding high-quality material[19], limited clinical computing skills or poor access to networked computers in the clinic or at the bedside. For a lucky few this will change soon with portable cellular Internet phones, if the limitations of battery life and screen size can be resolved. The benefits of their introduction throughout the National Health Service (NHS) will need to be studied rigorously in view of the high cost of the devices and the supporting infrastructure. A cheaper first stage would be to provide one or two suitable fixed computers in every clinic or ward. Sackett concluded from timing trials at the John Radcliffe hospital that clinicians could use a computer in a side-room to answer 16 questions in the time taken to consult a reserved machine in the library just four floors away[7].

Increasing emphasis on in-service training, clinical governance and the wider use of evidence, as well as the National Electronic Library of Health[20], means that every NHS ward, clinic or general practice will need ready access to a local computer offering information resources. It will be up to the medical profession to ensure that, subject to proven efficacy, this is followed by widespread adoption of portable devices, as foreseen a decade ago[21].

References

1   Funes M, Johnson N. *Honing your Knowledge Skills*. Oxford: Heinemann, 1998

2   Sackett D, Richardson WS, Rosenberg W, Haynes R. *Evidence Based Medicine*. London: Churchill Livingstone, 1997

3   Smith R. What clinical information do doctors need? *BMJ* 1996;**313**:1062–8

4   Ely JW, Osheroff JA, Ebell MH, Bergus GR, Levy BT, Chambliss ML, *et al.* Analysis of questions asked by family doctors regarding patient care. *BMJ* 1999;**319**:358–61

5   Gorman P, Helfand M. Information seeking in primary care: how physicians choose which clinical questions to pursue and which to leave unanswered. *Med Decis Making* 1995;**15**:113–19

6   Hersh W, Hickham DH. How well do physicians use electronic information retrieval systems? A framework for investigation and systematic review. *JAMA* 1998;**280**:1347–52

7   Sackett DL, Straus SE. Finding and applying evidence during clinical rounds: the 'evidence cart'. *JAMA* 1998;**280**:1336–8

8   Wyatt JC. Same information, different decisions: format counts. *BMJ* 1999;**318**:1501–2

9   Antman EM, Lau J, Kupelnick B, Mosteller F, Chalmers TC. A comparison of results of meta-analyses of randomized control trials and recommendations of clinical experts. *JAMA* 1992;**268**:240–8

10 Godlee F, Goldmann D, Donald A, Barton S, Wyatt J, Woolf S, eds. *Clinical Evidence*. London: BMJ Publishing, 1999 [http://www.clinicalevidence.org]

11 Wyatt JC, Vincent S. Selecting computer-based evidence sources. *Ann Oncol* 1999;**10**:267–73

12 Coiera E, Tombs V. Communication behaviours in a hospital setting: an observational study. *BMJ* 1998;**316**:673–6

13 Wyatt J. Use and sources of medical knowledge. *Lancet* 1991;**338**:1368–73

14 Hibble A, Kanka D, Pencheon D, Pooles F. Guidelines in general practice: the new Tower of Babel? *BMJ* 1998;**317**:862–3

15 Thomson R, McElroy H, Sudlow M. Guidelines on anticoagulant treatment in atrial fibrillation in Great Britain: variation in content and implications for treatment. *BMJ* 1998;**316**:509–13

16 Gorman P, Ash J, Wykoff L. Can primary care physicians' questions be answered using the medical literature? *Bull Med Lib Soc* 1994;**82**:140–6

17 Weed LL. New connections between medical knowledge and patient care. *BMJ* 1997;**315**:231–5

18 Johnson CG, Levenkron JC, Suchman AL, Manchester R. Does physician uncertainty affect patient satisfaction? *J Gen Intern Med* 1988;**3**:144–9

19 Wyatt JC. Measuring quality and impact of the World Wide Web. *BMJ* 1997;**314**:1879–81

20 Wyatt JC, Keen JR. The NHS's new information strategy. *BMJ* 1998;**317**:900

21 Wyatt J. Computer-based knowledge systems. *Lancet* 1991;**338**:1431–6

SECTION 1
IMPROVING YOUR CLINICAL KNOWLEDGE

2 Keeping up: continuing education or lifelong learning?

Biomedical knowledge doubles every 20 years[1] and clinical skills must constantly be updated. Yet, unless we are careful, our practice tends to fossilize after completion of formal professional training. How can this be avoided? There is no shortage of techniques to help clinicians improve their knowledge and skills right up to retirement[2]—face-to-face courses, speciality conferences, mailed educational materials, multimedia software, grand rounds, journal clubs, Internet sites, pharmaceutical company presentations. Complex schemes are run by colleges and deans to encourage participation (or, at least, attendance). The trouble is that, while traditional continuing education methods may increase our knowledge, they are less good at helping us apply this knowledge to clinical decisions or practice[3]. For example, Evans conducted a randomized study to assess the impact on clinical practice of a carefully designed information pack, known to improve knowledge about current management of hypertension, sent in 14 weekly instalments to Canadian doctors[4]. The intervention made no difference to the treatments that were used; in fact, the best predictor of doctors' decisions about antihypertensive treatment was their year of qualification, not whether they had been randomized to receive the information pack.

Improving clinical decisions and practice as well as knowledge

The assumption underlying traditional education is that the way knowledge enters the memory does not influence the ease with which it is later recalled and applied to decisions. This is incorrect: we now know that the problem-based approach is superior not only in improving memorization but also in aiding recall and application[2,5]. The problem-based learning (PBL) method entails waiting until the learner faces a decision or question, then providing access to the knowledge required for a response. The benefits of such active learning apply even if the clinical question or problem to be solved is simulated, as long as the learner becomes engaged in the dilemma. The efficacy of this approach is enhanced if learning takes place in the physical environment where the knowledge will be used. This is because our memory retrieves knowledge learned in the same context (e.g. the clinic) much more easily than facts learned in different contexts (the library or seminar room)[6].

The empirical psychological evidence about PBL makes sense: we learn lessons fastest and recall them most reliably when they originate from everyday experience. There is also good evidence that the method works in medicine. For example, 5–15 years after emerging from McMaster medical school (a pioneer in PBL), doctors showed greater understanding of current medical practice than did graduates from Toronto University (traditional)[7]. A systematic review indicated that, when rated by the supervising consultants, junior doctors trained by PBL methods scored more highly on clinical skills than did those with conventional training—though, interestingly, nurses rated the PBL graduates slightly lower[8].

So, for continuing medical education (CME), should we shift from conventional methods to PBL? What are the implications of such a move? The problem-based approach means finding solutions to clinical problems at the time they arise or soon after, with minimum effort. It means looking up the answer whenever we are unsure about what has happened or what to do. It means transforming CME from an intensive 2 hours a week (or a few days a year) to 1 minute here, 3 minutes there, prompted by the clinical problems and learning opportunities scattered through every working day. It emphasizes problem-solving and learning skills, such as how to find relevant answers fast—not the learning of facts. PBL is what we promise to do when we leave medial school but seldom achieve.

Difficulties with problem-based learning—and possible solutions

To achieve a shift towards PBL, the first thing is to recognize that we cannot get answers to every clinical problem or information need—especially since there are about two information needs for every three clinical encounters[9]. Many clinical information needs simply have no satisfactory answer, and some of the rest are better characterized as 'interesting questions' (see Chapter 1). Also, various practical difficulties arise when we try to pursue the PBL approach.

Too many questions, not enough time

What is the least time we should devote to keeping up to date, in an era when the human and economic impacts of clinical decisions, risk management and quality improvement are receiving ever closer attention? In my opinion, a reasonable investment would be 5–10% of our working life—i.e. 3–5 hours a week for the average doctor. However, UK Royal Colleges require only some 50 hours of formal CME *per year*—1 hour a week. This leaves a gap of 2–4 hours a week or 25–50 minutes a day between what will become mandatory and what seems reasonable.

The first strategy to square this circle is to adjust our threshold for seeking answers. Among relevant factors would be the degree of uncertainty, the likely clinical impact and the ease and speed of finding the answer[10]. Thus, the order of priorities for clinical impact would be:

1   Answers needed now, to inform a current decision or action

2   Answers needed before we next see the patient

3   Answers needed to guide the care of later patients or to reorganize clinical practice

4   Answers that interest us but have no obvious clinical implications.

When we have time, we can pursue all question categories. When under pressure, we can only pursue category 1 questions. However, if we never pursue other question categories, we will miss many clinical advances. Also, since one of the greatest challenges is to recognize where we lack knowledge, we ought sometimes to pursue questions even when we are only slightly uncertain of the answer.

A second strategy is to spend less time answering each question. This means gaining instant access to comprehensive, easily searched, knowledge resources.

The third strategy is to increase the time available for learning. Individually, we can work for longer hours, reserving time for 'reflective practice'. Sometimes this is easier when a colleague takes on the role of preceptor or mentor, exploiting 'teachable moments'[11] and perhaps writing us an educational prescription[12]. For the clinical profession, however, it means insistence on lifelong self-directed learning throughout every clinical career.

Lack of clear questions

Sometimes, in a moment of uncertainty, we neglect to formalize a question and then allow the matter to lapse. The solution is to encourage immediate identification of clinical questions. This is easy on ward rounds or when teaching students. When working alone some clinicians log their questions in a book and look up or discuss the answer with peers later. Structuring a question by deciding the kind of dilemma, the clinical goal, options being considered and relevant patient data (see Chapter 1) makes a question easier to recall and answer.

Some doctors tend to equate lack of knowledge with errors, believing that both are best forgotten. In a survey of 254 US medical residents questioned anonymously, 90% described making an error with a serious patient outcome. Only a little over half had discussed their mistakes with anyone. Those who had reported and discussed their error made more constructive changes in their clinical practice than those who had attributed the mistake to overwork[13]. If our routine clinical practice does not yield sufficient questions, then clinical audit and anonymous 'near miss' incident reports can provide rich seams to mine.

Lack of relevant, rigorous, usable answers

Questions are more easily asked than answered. What we need is a source of answers that are clinically relevant, scientifically sound and in a form that can influence decisions. Chapter 4 will discuss how to set up and run a small clinical library, close at hand and organized for rapid access. As much as possible of the material should be evidence-based and filtered for clinical relevance—for example, *Clinical Evidence*[14], the *Best Evidence* CD-ROM or a team library of journal articles (Chapter 3) focusing on systematic reviews[11]. In addition, a local medical library may be able to help with difficult questions by supplying Medline searches promptly (within 30 minutes) by e-mail or fax.

Telephone help lines have been provided for years by poisons and drug information services, providing instant answers to a restricted range of questions. Some libraries, primary care groups and academic departments are beginning to offer similar services with a broader range of topics, usually calling back or sending a summary or relevant article within 2 hours. Many of these services are underused and underfunded at present.

Parochialism

If the questions that you pursue are confined to your personal practice, you will become parochial; your knowledge and understanding will depend on the local casemix. To avoid this, consider participating in a multidisciplinary clinic or ward round, or network with colleagues via an e-mail discussion group. To widen their outlook, many clinicians read a general medical journal (Chapter 3) or look up points raised in replies to referrals, inpatient summaries, clinic letters or laboratory reports. And to make themselves ready for those rare serious events that require an instant response, some use high-fidelity patient simulators—for example, for management of cardiopulmonary arrest, anaesthetic accidents or brittle diabetes[15]. Commercial pilots can include time spent on simulators toward their mandatory continuing education, but this is not yet true of doctors.

Videoconferencing is another means to enhance in-service learning[16]. Telemedicine sessions offer the perfect opportunity for problem-based learning, with reserved time, one-to-one mentoring and a video of the consultation for participants to review later. Telemedicine projects often tail-off in their second or third year; one reason may be that knowledge and skills equilibrate within the group.

Lack of incentives

For some problem-based learners, the continuous expansion of personal knowledge will be sufficient exhilaration to sustain the effort; for rather more, the resolve to look up answers will wane as time goes by. One way to maintain momentum is to keep a running logbook of questions and answers; another is to conduct routine audits of clinical practice, comparing current results with those 6–12 months ago. Reducing the obstacles will help: it is much easier to look up a drug point in a 2-year-old *British National Formulary* in your desk drawer than to consult the current version in the practice library next door, let alone the postgraduate library 3 miles away with no car park. Electronic libraries and the Internet can bring the world's published work to your desktop but, as Ely found[10], they are at present slower than paper sources and yield fewer answers to clinical questions. This will soon change (Chapters 7–9).

A major incentive to learning is the opportunity to share insights. A short presentation often prompts enlightening discussion at weekly meetings, especially if it clearly defines the clinical dilemma and specifies the immediate sources searched, the answers found and the action taken. This activity can be formalized and shared as a 1-page 'critically appraised topic' (CAT)[12], and published on paper or a local intranet (Chapter 7).

Lack of recognition from professional organizations

The PBL approach, with its emphasis on individual, unsupervised and often undocumented learning, does not fit easily within the CME/postgraduate education allowance points system. Some colleges are moving towards recognizing self-directed learning. For example, since 1996 the Royal College of Physicians has included specially commissioned continuing-education material in every issue of its journal, and gives CME credits to those who return the associated self test. However, only 90 of the current circulation of 13 400 physicians currently return the self tests, of whom 65 get the necessary 80% to be awarded three CME points. The College also awards CME points to individuals who publish journal articles on relevant topics, but these must again be a small minority. The College is placing the CME articles and, perhaps more importantly, the self tests, on its website, setting a welcome precedent for recognizing reflective use of the Internet. However, it will be some time before

Table 2.1 Changes associated with problem-based lifelong learning

Old think	New think
Passively listening to lectures	Actively participating in learning sessions
Educator decides the topic	You decide the topic
You attend the CME courses and sessions you know most about	You actively seek out areas of ignorance and answers to your clinical dilemmas
Focus is on research results, pathophysiology, mechanisms	Focus is on what works in practice, what to do, problem solving
Reading a journal or textbook	Problem solving on real or simulated cases, answering a quiz, learning portfolio
Education to learn facts, pass exams	Learning to solve clinical problems, improve teamwork, clinical and information-seeking skills
Formal, timed courses	Informal, self-directed, on-the-job learning
Getting CME points for turning up	Getting points for participating, returning an MCQ, using learning materials, improving standards
Case presentation, journal club	Educational prescription, critically appraised topic, work on clinical simulator
Competition: keeping your knowledge to yourself	Sharing: open learning, exchange of knowledge and understanding to benefit patients and the health system
Knowledge belongs to the individual, so CME points accumulate to the individual	Communities of practice: learning is an attribute of the team and organization, and part of its quality and risk management strategies
Recertify the individual	Accredit the organization
Patients as passive recipients of care	Patients as sources of stimuli and as learning collaborators
Accept the learning curve: read about a new technique, practise it on patients	Reject the learning curve: work with an expert, perfect the technique on high fidelity models or simulators
Errors should be forgotten, hidden, denied	Errors are a learning experience, to be discussed and understood
Errors happen only to 'bad apples'	Errors happen to everyone

CME=Continuing medical education; MCQ=multi-choice questionnaire

the majority of clinicians use such a mechanism, and how can the scheme be extended to monitor and reward the learning that results from seeking answers to questions arising during individual clinical practice?

Conclusions

Taken as a whole, the shift away from continuing education implies a modest culture change (Table 2.1). Some of it has already taken place in undergraduate medical education and primary care, while clinical governance, risk management and the Information for Health strategy will further promote it.

Use of clinical questions to guide learning will always rely heavily on the motivation of individuals, teams and organizations, and goes hand in hand with a new open attitude to clinical errors and near misses. Motivation is especially necessary when it comes to funding the means to gain instant answers in clinical practice. Fortunately, electronic media will provide a simpler, cheaper and more up-to-date method for PBL than paper libraries, though more librarians will be needed to support them. Later I will discuss how to commission and use these.

References

1   Wyatt J. Use and sources of medical knowledge. *Lancet* 1991;**338**:1368–73

2   Wentz DK. Continuing medical education at a crossroads. *JAMA* 1990;**264**:18

3   Davis DA, Thomson MA, Oxman AD, Haynes RB. A systematic review of the effect of continuing medical education strategies. *JAMA* 1995;**274**:700–5

4   Evans CE, Haynes RB, Birkett NJ, *et al.* Does a mailed continuing education package improve physician performance? Results of a randomised trial. *JAMA* 1986;**255**:501–4

5   Schmidt HG, Norman GR, Boshuizen HPA. A cognitive perspective on medical expertise: theory and implications. *Acad Med* 1990;**65**:611–21

6   Lave J, Wenger E. *Situated Learning*. Cambridge: Cambridge University Press, 1991

7   Shin JH, Haynes RB, Johnston ME. Effect of problem-based, self directed undergraduate curriculum on life long learning. *Can Med Assoc J* 1993;**148**:969–76

8   Albanese MA, Mitchell S. Problem-based learning: a review of literature on its outcome and implementation issues. *Acad Med* 1993;**68**:52–81

9   Smith R. What clinical information do doctors need? *BMJ* 1996;**313**:1062–8

10   Ely J, Osheroff J, Ebell M, *et al.* Analysis of questions asked by family doctors regarding patient care. *BMJ* 1999;**319**:358–61

11   Badgett RG, O'Keefe M, Henderson MC. Using systematic reviews in clinical education. *Annals Intern Med* 1997;**126**:886–91

12   Sackett D, Richardson WS, Rosenberg W, Haynes R. *Evidence Based Medicine*. London: Churchill Livingstone, 1997

13   Wu AW, Folkman S, McPhee SJ, Lo B. Do house officers learn from their mistakes? *JAMA* 1991;**265**:2089–94

14   Godlee F, Goldmann D, Donald A, Barton S, Wyatt J, Woolf S, eds. *Clinical Evidence*. London: BMJ Publishing, 1999 [http://www.clinicalevidence.org]

15   Hovorka R, Andreassen S, Benn JJ, Olesen KG, Carson ER. Causal probabilistic network modelling—an illustration of its role in the management of chronic diseases. *IBM Systems J* 1992;**31**:635–48

16   Wallace S, Wyatt J, Taylor P. Telemedicine in the NHS for the millennium and beyond. *Postgrad Med J* 1998;**74**:721–8

3 Reading journals and monitoring current literature

The problem-based learning process described in the previous chapter—in which unresolved clinical questions generate searches for information as they arise—should help keep us ahead of the tidal wave of new data. However, ours would be a dull profession if we did not wish to broaden our knowledge beyond the current case mix. Moreover, patients can reasonably expect us to be well informed: the public takes a close interest in new clinical developments—in some parts of the USA half the people arriving for outpatient appointments carry an Internet print-out. Many journals now include news pages to help doctors keep up with information of this sort.

Keeping up

With what?

No one can keep up with the full ramifications of a single speciality, let alone the whole of medicine. Our goal should be to keep abreast of the knowledge most relevant to our responsibilities—clinical, teaching, research and administrative. The average general practitioner can get by with only a modest acquaintance with molecular biology, a clinical director of surgery with scant knowledge of dermatology. Laine suggests that we should each develop a personal mission statement embodying our professional goals, scope, and future plans, what we need to know and what we are happy to look up[1]. A mission statement must be realistic: start modestly and build from a successful base rather than risk disheartenment from the outset. An example for a radiologist with a special interest might be:

> *'My knowledge needs to be current in neuroradiology; I must be aware of general advances in radiology, other imaging methods and neurosurgery and know where to find more detail; I should have heard of other major medical developments'.*

How?

Other chapters in this book discuss the selection and use of books, multimedia, practice guidelines and continuing education methods; the previous chapter discussed the need to look up answers to *ad-hoc* clinical questions as part of lifelong learning. Each of these methods can provide a window on current knowledge. Here I deal specifically with regular journal-reading and the monitoring of publications by database-searching.

Reading journals

Regular reading

There are over 40 000 biomedical journals and the number doubles every 20 years[2]; we cannot hope to browse, let alone read, more than a tiny fraction. How should those few be selected?

The specialist primary biomedical journals are designed for researchers—scientist-to-scientist—not practising doctors[3]. The jobbing clinician should not take their content too seriously since they may well contain misleading pathophysiological insights or early clinical promises that will not be fulfilled. In many of the general medical and clinical speciality journals the editors take pains to select and publish material relevant to practising clinicians and give articles labels such as 'early report' and 'hypothesis' to make clear they differ from clinical articles and reviews. In choosing your journals, one criterion might be that the content should be peer reviewed; but this is an elastic term and offers no guarantee against poor material. A good policy is to avoid journals that commission every article published and those that depend wholly on advertisements for their income. Journal supplements sponsored by drug companies are commonly of low quality, and, if you are tempted to rely on journal articles and other materials distributed by drug or equipment companies, do not expect them to be unbiased[4]. To be indexed on Medline a journal must surmount various hurdles, so the quality is reasonable; at present there are 4000 of these.

In boiling the choice down to five or so, some journals are obvious. Most doctors will benefit from scanning one or more of the 'big four' general journals (*Lancet, BMJ, NEJM, JAMA*) plus a couple of major journals in their specialty such as *Gut* or the *British Journal of Surgery*. For the others, the choice may be determined by factors such as relevance of the articles to your work and the rigour with which they are presented[5]. But even if you subscribe to a journal, important articles are easily missed. This hazard is reduced by current awareness services. At local level, someone can photocopy and circulate the contents pages of journals most likely to interest colleagues and, more widely, a subscription to *Current Contents* can serve a similar purpose; some journals, such as the *BMJ* [www.bmj.com], will regularly e-mail their contents pages free of charge. Of course, tables of contents will give you only the titles of articles. More informative are the secondary or abstracting journals such as *Evidence Based Medicine*, *Evidence Based Mental Health* or *ACP Journal Club*. For each of these, a panel of clinicians scans hundreds of journals for articles with potential clinical impact which are then critically appraised. Even though coverage is restricted to clinical journals, the harvest is only 2–3% of all articles screened—a sobering comment on clinical research. Abstracts of the articles that survive the process are then reproduced or rewritten and an expert commentary is commissioned. As well as highlighting rigorous, clinically relevant results, these secondary journals often include useful editorials on methods for searching Medline or appraising articles, and a glossary of statistical methods and terms. They are thus an attractive way for working clinicians to obtain a distillate from a much wider range of journals than they could screen by themselves.

Which articles to read and act on

Your time is valuable, so, to decide which articles to read, why not apply basic critical appraisal methods? Start with relevance: if the study aim is either unclear or irrelevant to your mission, move on. A study is most likely to change your practice if it was conducted in a setting similar to your own, on a similar population, with endpoints you consider relevant. Next, consider whether the study results are likely to be correct. A basic criterion is whether the study design was appropriate to the question asked. It is not always true that 'evidence from randomised trials holds more weight than observational data'[1]: the best design for a study will depend on the question being asked[6]. For example, even a single case report may be highly convincing if it describes a rare but dangerous side-effect which disappeared when the drug was stopped and reappeared when treatment resumed. Finally, if the article is judged to describe the appropriate kind of study, is it free from the common biases that might threaten its validity? Checklists and explanations of these for various study types, and details of the critical appraisal process, are contained in Sackett's short and readable book[7] and in *JAMA*'s 'Reader's Guides' series.

Similar considerations apply to the electronic preprint articles found on servers such as PubMed Central or Netprints [www.clinmed.netprints.org]. The idea is that a copy of a paper is made available on the web before peer review[8]. Advantages of such preprints over their competitor, conference abstracts, are that they contain the full results, are more widely and rapidly accessible than conference proceedings, and allow feedback from readers. They may also allow negative studies to be reported and found more readily—for example, by people writing systematic reviews. However, since they are screened only for libel and breaches of patient confidentiality, not for quality or clinical relevance, clinicians should treat them with caution or await journal publication.

Doctors are rightly reluctant to act on a single small study and often wait for a review before changing their practice[1]. However, review articles of the traditional kind ('expert reviews') tend to use unspecified methods[9] which can be biased, and their conclusions lag many years behind primary studies[10]. A systematic review provides more reliable insights on a specific subject, such as the effectiveness of recombinant insulin in diabetes[7]. However, to guide a broader clinical decision such as which therapy to select for diabetes or how to keep up to date with the general management of diabetes, an expert review based on a systematic analysis of several large rigorous studies may be the best option.

How much to read

With time so short, there is a temptation to confine our scanning to abstracts or even article titles, but we should be very wary of this. Many titles promise much more than the study delivers, while some hide gems behind an inscrutable headline. Abstracts—especially structured abstracts—should tell us much more; however, when Pitkin compared the statements made in 264 structured abstracts in six major medical journals with the corresponding article, 20% of abstracts contained statements that were not substantiated in the article and 28% contained statements which disagreed with those in the article[11].

Rather than save time by reading abstracts alone, we need to schedule 1 or 2 hours a week to trace and obtain reading material. Once obtained it can be read later in odd gaps[1]. If we can identify where these gaps occur—between patients in the clinic, on the train to meetings, even *during* meetings—we can keep the reading material handy to fill them. However, we are more likely actually to read the material if it is relevant (which it will be if we follow the critical appraisal process) and if we have incentives. Incentives are again largely in our own hands. If we really want to read and keep up but need some external pressure to help us, we can arrange to give teaching sessions, promise patients that we will discuss a new therapy with them next time, or participate in a journal club.

Searching the published work

As well as browsing general and secondary journals and conducting searches to answer questions that arise in practice (Chapter 2), we can keep up by searching databases regularly. One suggestion is to develop a search strategy for a bibliographic database that coincides with your mission statement[1], perhaps adapting the published strategy from a relevant Cochrane systematic review. Your strategy may take a while to develop and refine, even with a librarian to help. However, once developed it can be stored and re-run monthly to yield all new material in minutes. Even with the best search strategy, some articles will prove irrelevant; one way to filter them out is to review abstracts on screen before ordering the full text.

Which bibliographic database?

There are at least 10 commonly used bibliographic databases or routes to them, with differing characteristics. In addition, several of the secondary journals are available electronically (Appendix 3.1); for definitions of terms see Ref. 12. Most clinicians start with Medline, but HealthStar (quality improvement), Psychlit (mental health) and Cancerlit (cancer) are others that may be useful.

Should I do it myself, ask a librarian or adapt an existing strategy?

Nowadays most clinicians will perform their own free-form searches. However, in a study of 158 clinicians given a 3-hour Medline training session, Medline novices were only able to locate 45% of relevant articles, and 70% of all the articles they identified were judged irrelevant[13]. Corresponding figures for Medline-experienced clinicians were 50% and 57% while for librarians they were 53% and 38%. Medline experience does substantially reduce the amount of irrelevant material retrieved but only slightly improves the percentage of relevant articles located.

For further improvement, we must combine a stored, tried and tested search strategy with a few keywords tailored to our needs. Thus, if your interest is in randomized trials of a named drug, the PubMed Clinical search filter [www.ncbi.nlm.nih.gov/PubMed] for therapy will find 99% of all trials and 74% of the articles it locates should prove relevant. If the 26% irrelevant articles trouble you, you can choose a search strategy with a 3% irrelevance rate (97% specific), but this retrieves only 57% of all the correct studies[14]. Similar search strategies are available to identify rigorous studies relevant to diagnosis, aetiology or prognosis.

The decision to devise your own searches, use PubMed's ready-made clinical queries or ask a librarian depends on whether your question is confined to therapy, diagnosis, aetiology or prognosis (favouring a PubMed clinical query), concerns other issues but is well formulated (a general PubMed query) or fuzzy (you may need a librarian to help you formulate the search). It also depends on how much time you have to browse the search results on screen and refine your search strategy accordingly. A useful method when the database's controlled vocabulary is patchy or variably applied by indexers—such as in medical informatics—is to start with a known target paper and discover how it has been indexed. Citation searches (looking for articles that refer to a known classic paper) can also help. A final option is to call or e-mail a question-answering service, in which you refine the question with a librarian or information scientist.

Organizing reprints

Once we identify a promising article, we need to obtain the full text. Conventional document delivery services charge up to £6 ($10) per article and take from 3 to 10 days. Sometimes our local library will fax us a copy in an hour for free. If our institution has a licence to online full text of the right journal, or the article appeared in the handful of public-spirited journals such as the *BMJ* that allow full-text access to all, we can print out an electronic clone of the original.

Even in this electronic age, paper copies of articles are useful because they remind us to read them, can be browsed unobtrusively on the train or during meetings, can be annotated, can be filed as a reminder in relevant patients' notes, and can be read 40% faster than on screen. However, if we are ever to find them again, we need a system.

In view of the way most doctors work, any reprint filing system must be designed to make the filing and retrieval of articles trivially easy. Simplest perhaps is a row of open labelled magazine files, one per clinical topic, to which current articles are always added on the right hand side and so automatically kept in year order. Brightly coloured A4 cards can be added to each file to celebrate New Year and facilitate navigation. Alternative systems that require more upkeep include a hanging file for each detailed topic arranged alphabetically, and files containing numbered articles with a computer keyword index[15]. Scanning of each article into a computerized document management system is also possible but requires time, dedication and cash—and may even tempt some writers into plagiarism.

Conclusion

Keeping up is painful because it means learning new insights, relearning old insights and forgetting outdated insights[1]. Targeted reading of articles in paper journals and identifying new articles through bibliographic systems takes time and effort. As with other lifelong learning approaches, it may be worth collaborating with colleagues to share out the work and the resulting discoveries. However, although many doctors value the social pressure of regular meetings such as journal clubs, careful planning is needed to determine the scope, who will do which searches, and which strategies should be used.

References

1   Laine C, Wenberg DS. How can physicians keep up to date? *Annu Rev Med* 1999;**50**:99–110

2   Wyatt J. Use and sources of medical knowledge. *Lancet* 1991;**338**:1368–73

3   Haynes RB. Loose connections between peer-reviewed clinical journals and clinical practice. *Ann Intern Med* 1990;**113**:724–8

4   Stryer D, Bero L. Characteristics of material distributed by drug companies. *J Gen Intern Med* 1996;**11**:575–83

5   Haynes RB, McKibbon KA, Fitzgerald D, Guyatt GH, Walker CJ, Sackett DL. How to keep up with the medical literature: deciding which journals to read regularly. *Ann Intern Med* 1986;**105**:309–12

6   Sackett DL, Wennberg JE. Choosing the best research design for each question. *BMJ* 1997;**315**:1636

7   Sackett D, Richardson WS, Rosenberg W, Haynes R. *Evidence Based Medicine.* London: Churchill Livingstone, 1997

8   Delamothe T, Smith R, Keller MA, Sack J, Witscher B. Netprints: the next phase in the evolution of biomedical publishing. *BMJ* 1999;**319**:1515–16

9   Bramwell VH, Williams CJ. Do authors of review articles use systematic methods to identify, assess and synthesise information? *Ann Oncol* 1997;**8**:1185–95

10 Antman EM, Lau J, Kupelnick B, Mosteller F, Chalmers TC. A comparison of results of meta-analyses of randomized control trials and recommendations of clinical experts. *JAMA* 1992;**268**:240–8

11 Pitkin RM, Branagan MA, Burmeister LF. Accuracy of data in abstracts of published research articles. *JAMA* 1999;**281**:1110–11

12 Wyatt JC, Vincent S. Selecting computer-based evidence sources. *Ann Oncol* 1999;**10**:267–73

13 McKibbon KA, Haynes RB, Walker Dilks CJ, *et al.* How good are clinical Medline searches? A comparative study of end-user and librarian searches. *Comp Biomed Res* 1990;**23**:583–93

14 Haynes RB, Wilczynski N, McKibbon KA, Walker CJ, Sinclair JC. Developing optimal search strategies for detecting clinically sound studies in MEDLINE. *J Am Med Informatics Assoc* 1994;**1**:447–58

15 Haynes RB, McKibbon KA, Fitzgerald D, Guyatt GH, Walker CJ, Sackett DL. How to keep up with the medical literature: how to store and retrieve articles worth keeping. *Ann Intern Med* 1986;**105**:978–84

Appendix 3.1 Characteristics of some frequently used bibliographic databases and secondary electronic resources

Database name (publisher)	Medium	Main contents	Source of data	Clinical speciality	First item	Update frequency	Size	Quality assurance	Coded fields
Bandolier (Oxford NHS R&D Directorate)	Web and print	Commentaries on rigorous clinically relevant published SRs and 1° studies, articles on EBM	All types	All	1994	1 month	c. 400 articles		No
Best Evidence (ACP)	CD-ROM	Structured abstracts & commentaries on rigorous, clinically relevant SRs and 1° studies	All types, from ACP J Club (1991 on) and EBM J (1995 on)—scan 90 journals	All	1991	3 months	1100 abstracts, commentaries	All studies passed ACP critical appraisal criteria	No
CancerLit (NCI)	CD-ROM InterNet	Bibliographic	All types	Oncology	Some journals from 1963 rest 1976–	1 month	1.3 million	Medline+some journal articles; some monographs, proceedings	some other MeSH, etc
Clinical Evidence (*BMJ*)	CD-ROM intranet	Systematic reviews	RCTs and epid studies	All		6 months	400 topics, growing	Own criteria+peer review	
Cochrane Database of Systematic Reviews (Cochrane)	CD-ROM (abstracts free on Web)	Cochrane systematic reviews	Published and unpublished RCTs	All	1994	3 months	550 SRs, growing	Cochrane SRs only	MeSH coded
EMBase (Elsevier)	CD-ROM intranet	Bibliographic; abstracts on 80%	All types	All—especially pharmaceutical info	1980	15 days	7 million documents from 4000 journals	Original journal articles; some monographs, letters, conference proceedings	c. 25
HealthStar (NLM)	Web	Bibliographic; abstracts	All types	Health services research, admin	1975	1 week	3 million	Original journal articles; some monographs, proceedings	MeSH coded, c. 25
Medline (Ovid, Silver Platter)	CD-ROM intranet	Bibliographic; abstracts on most	All types	All	1966	1–4 weeks	9 million documents from 4300 journals	Original journal articles, some monographs, proceedings	22
Medline (PubMed, NCBI)	Web	Bibliographic; abstracts on most	All types	All	1966	Daily for pre-Medline, weekly for rest	9 million documents from 4300 journals	Anything in journals, inc. letters; 'Clinical Queries' apply quality fillers	c 25
PsychLit (Am Psych Assoc; Ovid, Aries, etc.)	CD-ROM	Bibliographic; abstracts on most	All types	Psychology and mental health	1987	3 months	1.2 million from 1300 journals	Original articles; some monographs, proceedings	No

ACP= American College of Physicians; NCI=National Cancer Institute; NLM=National Library of Medicine; NCBI=National Center for Biotechnology Information; EBM=evidence-based medicine; SR=systematic review; RCT=randomized controlled trial; MeSH=medical subject headings

4 Books and multimedia as reference material*

Most medical practices, clinical departments and health organizations maintain a collection of reference materials, whether just a few volumes on a shelf or a carefully managed library or information service. Medical librarians will usually say that, given proper institutional recognition and revenue support, they could greatly improve the content and presentation of their collection. Journals are particularly expensive and need to be carefully selected and were discussed in Chapter 3. Here, we consider two other kinds of reference material—books and multimedia, the latter accessed either on compact disk or on the World Wide Web.

What kind of reference material to buy or recommend

A local benefactor gives you £50 000 to restock your postgraduate library. Should you invest in books and shelves, or in computers and multimedia packages?

Table 4.1 compares the key characteristics of the three kinds of reference material considered here. The familiar book format still has some clear advantages—for instance, portability, no need for special equipment, ease of reading and generally high quality content. Drawbacks of bound paper are its bulk, the difficulties of manual searching and of sharing content without additional copies, the inability to update material, and high cost per volume. The ready portability of books is a disadvantage as well as an advantage: they are easily lost or stolen.

Electronic media can be searched more quickly and are easier to share and update; consequently they are more current and cheaper per reader than paper. However, since a computer is needed they are less portable than books and take longer to read—40% longer on screen than on paper[1]. The relative cheapness of CD or Web publishing also means that the quality of electronic material tends to be lower than that of printed material—and some Web material is a triumph of form over content[2]. Also, local technical support is necessary for the different types of material and the computers through which they are accessed, and many readers require training before they can use an electronic resource. Electronic material does

---

*With some material by Betsy Anagnostelis, Librarian, Royal Free Hospital, London, UK

Table 4.1 Characteristics of print, compact disk and World Wide Web reference material

	Print format	Compact disk	World Wide Web
Cost per item	£20–£200 once	£50–£250 once or per annum	Nil–£250 per year
Bulk and weight	Medium–high	Low	Not applicable
Portability	Medium	Low (notebook PC needed)	Low (notebook PC needed)
Equipment needed	Nil	Stand-alone PC ($\pm$printer)	Networked PC ($\pm$printer)
Training needed	No	Yes	Yes
Tailoring to user needs	Slightly: highlight, annotate	Usually—track recent history; bookmark, annotate	Yes—bookmark, recent history
Ease of reading	High	Low	Low
Ease of searching	Low	High	Medium
Ease of sharing	Low; zero if tailored	Medium if networked	High
Interactive	No	Often	Often
Updating method	New book	New CD	Not applicable—users access a central information resource
Currency of content	Low	Medium	Medium–high
Quality of content	Medium–high	Medium–high	Varies: very poor–high
Security	Low—easily removed	Low to medium: CD readily accessed from stand-alone PC; less readily removed from networked PC	High: users access the central information resource

offer new possibilities such as interactivity, the inclusion of audio and video clips and tailoring to an individual reader's needs or preferences. Interactive characteristics such as these are explored in the final section of this chapter and also in Chapters 7 and 9. Printed material still forms the foundation of any core collection.

How to choose books for a core collection

The orthopaedics team requests a multivolume atlas and an operative procedure manual costing £1500. The neurosurgeons, and then the neuroradiologists, respond with similar demands

Books are expensive and journals even more so. Some libraries use informal criteria to prioritize purchases, such as the opinion of the library committee on whether the work comes within the scope of the collection. Others set explicit criteria for selecting material and stick to these whatever the pressure. One such might be the frequency of use of the previous edition or of similar works in the library, assessed from the lending records or from reshelving studies (in-library readers are asked to leave all material on the desks after consultation, for recording before reshelving[3]). One cannot, however, know the frequency of use of a book not yet bought, and there may be nothing like it in the library. Furthermore, even time-consuming measures such as date-stamping of each in-library use seem to underestimate actual use[3].

What other criteria might be applied? One is the reputation of the author, editor, series editor or publisher: an informal short cut is to peruse the information on the dust jacket. A more objective approach is to measure the response of other authors or independent critics in terms of citations, but this is slow and reflects only the extent to which the work is cited in published articles[4]. An alternative is to look at independent book reviews; when there is consensus among reviewers, this is helpful. A more indirect measure of the opinions of others is the longevity of the work, measured by the number of editions it has been through. The drawback is that this excludes good new books in an established area and all books in a new area. If local opinion is key, an informal panel of 5–10 target readers can request the local bookshop to send all the books on the shortlist on approval, those not selected to be returned. This method is best reserved for very expensive works or occasions when multiple copies are to be bought, for example by students. Bookshops are increasingly reluctant to provide material on approval.

As well as these indirect criteria, the decision whether or not to purchase a book will be influenced by intrinsic characteristics. Here are some examples:

- Whether it contains information of immediate importance not readily available elsewhere (e.g. poison antidotes for an A&E library)
- Style: narrative textbooks might receive lower priority than reference books (e.g. a pharmacopoeia, *Clinical Evidence*, the *Medical Directory*), methods books (e.g. about the principles of clinical examination, interpreting laboratory results, setting up an audit programme) or books designed to help those revising for specific exams
- Scope: a textbook providing broad coverage may be preferred to one that focuses on a single disease
- Frequency of the disorder addressed: a monograph about diabetes might take priority over one on Pendred's syndrome
- Durability of content: a book with enduring content is worth more than one likely to be outdated soon

- Cost, or cost per page: any continuing commitment, such as time required to file updates in a loose-leaf volume and annual subscription, needs to be taken into account
- Adequacy of the index, figures, tables and overall organization of the work.

A planned approach to development of a collection demands knowledge of the needs of the users and institutions served. What are the areas on which to concentrate resources? Referral to a library committee is usual, but can be slow and inefficient. There is much to be said for using library liaison officers who can offer a quick opinion on the quality of potential purchases and provide greater continuity.

When determining your priorities and collection policy, it is wise to avoid overlap with other local libraries. Sometimes a reciprocal agreement can be made.

How to choose a multimedia package

Doctors in training ask for a new range of multimedia packages to be purchased, to complement the book collection. The librarian now regrets the £6000 he spent on multimedia 2 years ago, already obsolete

Multimedia packages, with their full-motion video, dramatic music and digitized sounds, can be very seductive. As with computer games, the potential purchaser is commonly offered a 5-minute demonstration carefully crafted to impress, while the accuracy, detail and presentation of the main content may be less inspiring. With a book one turns quickly from the dust jacket to sample the main content by perusing the index, checking the table of contents and browsing the pages. With software it is hard to sample the main content without first learning how it is organized and how to navigate. Navigation methods differ from package to package or even between versions of the same package. Some multimedia packages get round such difficulties by including a clickable graphic map of the contents. The use of standard Web browser software, even if the content is distributed on a CD-ROM, helps users to navigate in a standard way. This also allows the user to explore associated live material online—for example, updated content, simulations or linked websites (see Chapters 7 and 8).

Many of the criteria for evaluating books apply to multimedia packages but there are some additional issues to consider[5]. Presentation of content is a key element. For example, content needs to be presented in easily digested modules appropriate to the medium, rather than merely as a screen view of a book. Readers with different professional backgrounds should be able to choose different paths through the material and to use the material in different ways— for example, as a dictionary, as a reference or tutorial resource, or to answer self-tests.

Ideally, the content should include non-text material such as moving images, audio, interactive quizzes and simulations of normal or deranged physiology. The content should be up to date and there should be provision for regular revision.

Users differ in their preferences for accessing computer applications and this diversity should be catered for by allowing alternative ways to issue commands—for example, by clicking on buttons or selecting from menus[6]. Personal preferences for screen layout, navigation method and printing can similarly be respected, and the package should be sharable across computer networks, looking the same on different types of computer. A tutorial for users should be included. The cost of a single or institution-wide licence, support and regular updates should be reasonable in relation to the content and function offered. Finally, the package should work on the computers currently available, not force the institution into an expensive upgrade programme.

How to catalogue, organize and secure a library

No one can find the new books you bought only 3 months ago. Are they just mis-shelved or on loan and, if so, to whom?

A medical library of only 200 volumes represents an asset of over 5000. To ensure that users can find the material they need, every collection of more than a few dozen volumes needs to be catalogued so that items can be retrieved, classified so that items on similar subjects are physically adjacent, and indexed to enhance subject-based retrieval. To do these effectively requires special skills and knowledge. The National Library of Medicine (NLM) classification scheme is widely used by medical libraries, and the NLM works hard to keep the scheme up to date. For subjects related to medicine, such as sociology and education, many medical libraries employ the Library of Congress (LC) scheme, since the NLM classification is a specially developed section of the LC classification.

Subject indexing can present its own set of problems. What words should we use to describe an orthopaedic atlas or an audit manual? For consistency you need a controlled vocabulary or thesaurus of terms, and there is much to be said for the Medical Subject Headings (MeSH) used in Medline, revised and reissued annually. Retrieval is enhanced if several subject headings are assigned to each volume to reflect the breadth of coverage. The catalogue can be made available both inside the library and remotely by use of Web technology (see Chapter 8). Additions to the collection can be publicized in a library newsletter or by e-mail to library users.

What about security? This is increasingly troublesome in both small and large libraries. The first step is to clarify who is authorized to use the collection: although a library may be open to all for reference, loans can reasonably be restricted to registered members. The second step is to ensure that all stock is identifiable. All books need to be stamped in at least three places. It is advisable to designate a reference section and to ensure that all reference books are clearly marked on the spine. If the library contains a substantial amount of material that is not for loan, put a photocopier on the premises. This avoids ambiguity if someone is found with reference-only material outside the library. If loans are allowed they need to be tracked, together with book returns. For sizeable collections, the practical way to do this is with library automation software. Access control systems may also be necessary if stock is being lost. Measures such as these will help to slow the depreciation rate of the collection and increase the speed and accuracy of searches for relevant material.

References

1   Wyatt JC, Wright P. Medical records 1: design should help use of patient data. *Lancet* 1998;**352**:1375–8

2   Wyatt JC. Measuring quality and impact of the World Wide Web. *BMJ* 1997;**314**:1879–81

3   Harris C. A comparison of issues and in-library use of books. *Aslib Proc* 1977;**29**:118–26

4   Institute of Scientific Information. Cited reference searching: an introduction. [www.isinet.com/training/jobaids/citerefpr/prim1.html]

5   Wyatt J. Evaluating electronic consumer health material. *BMJ* 2000;**320**:159–60

6   Wright P, Lickorish A. Menus and memory load: navigation strategies in interactive search tasks. *Int J Human-Computer Stud* 1994;**40**:965–1008

SECTION 2
HELPING PATIENTS AND PEERS TO CHANGE

5 Improving information for patients

All over the world, governments are pressing the notion that health is an individual responsibility. The public, patients and carers are being urged to learn about preventive care and to use informal support except when health services are essential[1]. In the UK, the National Health Service invested heavily in the freephone Health Information Service, and this was rapidly eclipsed by NHSDirect. Many drugs have undergone transition from licensed to over-the-counter use; and a new initiative, UK Online, provides government information in a manner designed for the needs of the citizen—for example, a website focused on life episodes such as having a baby. The motive is citizen empowerment, and the aim is not just to inform patients and carers but also to engage them in health decisions.

This global trend coincides with a remarkable growth of technologies for communicating with the public. For example, 37% of the UK public already have access to the web, and the figure will be 50% by the end of 2000. Over 20 million mobile phones in the UK can already receive SMS text messages, and third-generation mobile Internet phones will replace the restricted WAP phones. The Government has put money into development of health applications for interactive digital TV; and patient-held records, being considered as part of the NHS modernization agenda, could also increase the demand for health knowledge.

However, different people have different coping styles. Some patients want to know everything and express strong opinions on the choice of procedure or possible outcomes; others are happier not knowing the full facts, preferring to leave the decisions to their doctor. Although, in a consultation, individual coping strategies must be taken into account, in general we can predict several benefits from giving patients greater access to clinical knowledge. First, it may reduce anxiety, particularly if the patient or carer has a misconception that we can correct. Second, understanding of risk factors, preventive care or self care (such as how to recognize when things are getting worse) may lead to less disease, earlier presentation of disease or more appropriate use of health services. Third, information may improve a patient's appointment-keeping and adherence to therapy. For example, one study revealed that twice as many discharged patients knew about their drugs and brought them to follow-up appointments when they were given an information leaflet about their therapy[2]. However, a systematic review[3] of 13 randomized trials indicates that information alone does not improve adherence; it has to be part of a package of measures. Finally, shared decision-making ought to make professional practice more interesting, lead to better tailoring of management to individual patient preferences, and improve health outcomes.

Informing the public or patients

Three broad methods for informing the public are:

- Decision aids, which provide individual patients with information about their symptoms, drugs, or the options they face; these may also contain information on the disease and probabilities of alternative outcomes
- Planned mass media campaigns targeted at groups, not individuals
- Uncoordinated media coverage of topical health issues.

Sometimes patient information can be very effective. For example, in a small Danish randomized trial, patients who were told that their chronic chest complaint was 'smoker's lung' were twice as likely as controls to have stopped smoking 1 year later[4]. In another randomized study, a leaflet informing patients about the aetiology and natural course of viral upper respiratory tract infections significantly reduced general practice reattendance rates[5]. A systematic review identified 17 randomized trials of such individual patient decision aids[6]. Overall, the information produced better knowledge of options and outcomes, lower conflict scores and more active patient participation in decisions, without an increase in anxiety (but also without an increase in satisfaction with the decisions). The extra information had a variable effect on patients' decisions, ranging from a 26% reduction in willingness to undergo major surgery to no effect on decisions about screening tests or circumcision of a baby son. Complex decision support tools such as computer-based multimedia or video were only slightly better at reducing decisional conflict and led to slightly higher knowledge scores than simpler ones. This is consistent with recent work in Cardiff showing that, for decision-making about hormone replacement therapy, asthma and fetal screening for Down syndrome, video is no better than a well-designed patient information leaflet based on the video transcript (Wright P, personal communication).

What about mass media? A Cochrane systematic review found no randomized trials but identified 17 rigorous time-series studies of effects of mass media on health service utilization[7]. Fourteen were studies of formal media campaigns lasting from 1 week to 4 years, while the remaining three studied unplanned media coverage of specific health issues. Sixteen of the studies were reported as positive but reanalysis showed that only seven demonstrated a statistically significant impact on health service utilization. The overall impact of the 14 planned campaigns on health service utilization was a 54% change in the intended direction (either reduction of inappropriate use or increase in underused services), while unplanned media coverage led to a 24% change, about half as effective. The effectiveness also varied according to the kind of health service utilization targeted, with a 96% increase in immunization rates (pooled results from two studies), a 12% increase in cancer screening (seven studies), a 42% increase in HIV testing (three studies) and a 45% increase in the use of emergency services for myocardial infarction (two studies).

Potential drawbacks of informing patients

Some clinicians declare that 'a little learning is a dang'rous thing', expressing concerns that include:

- Creating a nation of worried well or 'cyberchondriacs'
- Dehumanizing the doctor–patient relationship by shifting information-giving from the clinical encounter to telephone or Internet
- Prolonging clinical encounters because patients have more questions, and doctors may need to counter Internet-borne rumours
- Information providers trying to manipulate the public to suit their own ends.

Arguments against these propositions are that patients with chronic diseases have more time and motivation than anyone else to inform themselves about their condition. In middle-class areas one in six patients has either trained in a health profession or has a close relative who has trained, so may expect detailed information. The last point, about manipulation, may be true, but most people know they should be sceptical about product claims.

There does exist a strong desire for information. In a survey of 250 cancer patients, 80% wanted as much information as possible; 96% wanted to know if they had cancer and 91% the chance of cure[8]. Women, patients younger than 65, patients treated radically and those from more affluent areas were more likely to want information about possible treatment options.

Thus, the aim must now be to push ahead while doing our best to limit the drawbacks.

What do patients want to know?

There is a huge range of information that people might wish to have—ranging from 'I wonder if I should lose weight' to the harrowing 'Should I let this surgeon correct my baby's transposition?'. This book concerns health knowledge so we will not discuss here the question of providing public access to professional performance data, though the NHS Information Strategy asserts the importance of this[9]. Nor will we consider information about the NHS (e.g. where is the nearest dermatology clinic?), obtaining contact details or getting support (I'd like to talk to someone else with psoriasis).

With its low cost and widely known telephone number, the NHSDirect helpline provides excellent insights into the kind of health questions to which the public want answers. Analysis and coding of transcripts of 267 randomly selected calls from June 1999 revealed that the main topic was patient complaints or symptoms in 72%, diagnoses or diseases in 22%, diagnostic, screening or preventive procedures in 5% and medication or treatment in 1%[10]. The calls were further classified by the body system concerned—see Table 5.1.

Table 5.1   Main topic of 267 randomly selected calls to
NHSDirect, June 1999, classified by body system.
[Data from Munro (Ref 10)]

Classification	%
Unspecified	20
Digestive	17
Musculoskeletal	15
Skin	14
Respiratory	9
Neurological	8
Eye	4
Ear	2.3
Social problem	2.3
Male genital	2
Urological	1.5
Circulatory	1
Psychological	1
Endocrine/metabolic/nutrition	1
Pregnancy, family planning	0.8
Female genital	0.8

One surprise was the rarity of requests for information about circulatory troubles; this may reflect public preconceptions about the urgency of such disorders or the role of NHSDirect.

Where do patients currently go for information?

It is hard to know exactly where patients learn what they know about health. Pupils are taught about personal health at school, people buy 'home doctor' books, and there are daily health programmes on radio and TV and articles in newspapers and magazines. The 1990s saw the advent of whole magazines devoted to men's health. However, the impact of these media on the public's knowledge of the structure and function of the body is unclear. In one study, 65% of surgical patients gave completely wrong answers about the function of internal organs and 58% placed organs in the wrong position on a body chart[11]. Presumably, their knowledge about abnormal function was even more sketchy.

One contemporary indication of where people turn for health advice is a survey of 15 000 randomly selected people in the catchment areas of the three first-wave NHSDirect sites

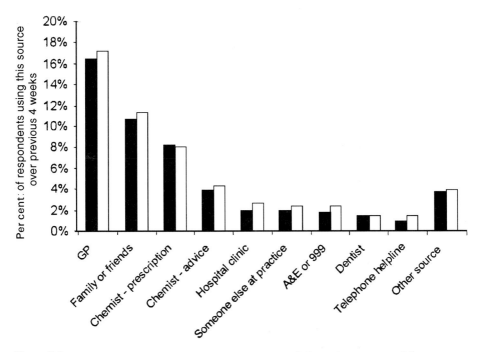

Figure 5.1 **Sources of unplanned advice or treatment in people in catchment areas of first-wave NHSDirect sites.** ■ **1998;** □ **1999.** [Data from Munro (Ref 10)]

conducted just before the helpline was set up in 1998 and repeated 1 year later[10]. Responses came from 70% with features typical of the UK adult population. In the 4 weeks before the survey, 38% of respondents had sought help or advice for a health problem (unchanged after NHSDirect was implemented). Figure 5.1 shows the overall rates of unplanned use of the main sources of health advice or treatment.

After GPs (17%) and high-street chemists (total 12%), family or friends (11%) are the commonest single source, with all others accounting together for only 12%. However, if family and friends use the Internet, this may become an equally useful way to reach patients.

Key issues relevant to patient information

Quality

One major concern with certain media, especially Internet websites, is the variable quality of information, which may be incomplete, badly organized or inaccurate[12]; such deficiencies can have serious consequences[13]. This leads on to how doctors should respond when a patient offers a web printout. A check on the date of preparation, sources used, qualifications of the author and who is sponsoring the site should help to establish the likely accuracy of the information presented. Looking for a quality label such as that issued by Health on the Net foundation [www.hon.ch] may help separate wheat from chaff. Some websites act as portals, appraising other sites according to explicit criteria; OMNI is an excellent example [www.omni.ac.uk]. The Discern checklist helps in the scoring of how closely material is based on evidence—but few sources do well on this score [www.discern.org]. The NHSDirect online site [www.nhsdirect.nhs.uk] uses this approach but also provides other material which does not yet approach the Discern standard; it is very popular, with about 100 000 hits a day. Finally, patients can be referred to an excellent website that logs quackery: [www.quackwatch.com].

Choosing appropriate media

We tend to think of patient information as leaflets, but a key issue is to avoid social exclusion and enhance accessibility. Thus, information may need to be translated to other languages and made available in alternative media—including audiotapes (such as the College of Health phone lines) or videotape for those with limited reading skills (up to a quarter of the adult population), large print for visually impaired people and Braille for deaf–blind people[14]. Brevity, visually attractiveness and simplicity are also key elements. Public kiosks that allow privacy but make information available in shopping centres or libraries have a clear role, but

Box 5.1   Effective writing for patients (adapted from Ref 15)

- Place the most important information first or last
- Write in a conversational style with short words and sentences
- Limit each paragraph to a single message
- Focus on specific personal experiences rather than generalities
- Ensure that the use of words is consistent
- Use headers to alert readers to what is coming
- Cut out irrelevant information
- In general, write in positive sentences
- Use negative sentences when advising patients to avoid actions
- Ask patients to read your draft and to suggest how to improve it

can be bulky and expensive and need to be further evaluated. Some patients or carers are so bewildered they do not even know where to start. A charity called Start Here acts as a pathfinder to this group.

Assessing readability

The best way to assess readability is to ask patients for their opinions; for research purposes this can be quantified by getting them to fill in missing words in material they have previously read—the Cloze technique[15]. Computed readability measures such as the Gunning Fogg index (accessible under document statistics in some wordprocessors) can be a useful guide but may not be accurate, particularly in chronic diseases where patients become familiar with medical jargon[15]. The ultimate test of patient materials is their impact on actual patient decisions, actions and outcomes, but few studies have been performed[16].

Improving readability

No medium will be effective unless patients can readily find and interpret the information it contains. Mayberry *et al.* have summarized 'information design' principles based on sound empirical findings[17], in their paper on effective writing for patients[15]—see Box 5.1.

One particular difficulty in communicating with the public concerns the matter of risk—as politicians know to their cost. A classic example is the 1995 media scare about the doubling of venous thromboembolism rates with third-generation oral contraceptives, which led to a substantial rise in unplanned pregnancies. Had the rarity of the side-effect (the baseline rate was only 75 per million) and the high proportion of women not developing it (99.99%) been emphasized, it is doubtful that the public would have overreacted in this way. Thus, the language used to communicate risk to the press or public requires scrupulous attention.

Avoiding unnecessary complexity

The cost of multimedia or video is rarely justified except to address specific impairments—because, as I pointed out earlier, they seem no better at informing or alleviating anxiety than a well-designed printed leaflet with the same content. An example of this is a trial comparing uptake of fetal anomaly scans in antenatal patients exposed to a sophisticated touch-screen computer system costing 25 000, or a leaflet, in a Scottish clinic: the scan rate was only 7% higher in the touch-screen group[18]. Equally, there is interest in tailoring information to the individual by asking the patient some questions first or linking to electronic patient records. While elegantly tailored smoking-cessation and other leaflets can be generated, their contribution to better informed patient choice is unclear.

Conclusions

At present we do not involve patients sufficiently in decisions about their own health. An exhaustive study of 1057 taped encounters with 59 US primary-care physicians and 65 surgeons showed that only 9% of the decisions were adequately informed, even though the average encounter lasted 16.5 minutes, double that in the UK[19]. Although surgical encounters were 3 minutes shorter, those decisions were better informed, so lack of time may not be the issue.

Communication about health with patients and the public is a growth industry, and the medical profession should engage in it. There are some good materials available and we should always strive to avoid reinvention; however, when the quality of existing material is imperfect, the best solution may be to write our own—perhaps with the aid of someone familiar with writing for the public, for example a friendly journalist, and patients themselves. Modern technology can also help: the half-empty rack of dog-eared leaflets in our surgery could be replaced by new printouts from an evidence-based website such as [www.patient.co.uk] (which, despite its commercial sounding title, is run by two Newcastle GPs). This avoids the need for stock control, and we can even e-mail patients with a pointer to the website, allowing them to check for updates themselves. This is a perfect way to respond to the increasing number of patient e-mail requests for information[20].

References

1   Smith R. The future of health care systems. *BMJ* 1997;**314**:1495–6

2   Sandler DA, Mitchell JRA, Fellows A, Garner ST. Is an information booklet for patients leaving hospital helpful and useful? *BMJ* 1989;**298**:870–4

3   Haynes RB, McKibbon KA, Kanani R. Systematic review of randomised trials of interventions to assist patients to follow prescriptions for medications. *Lancet* 1996;**348**:383–6

4   Brandt CJ, Ellegard H, Jeonsen M, Kallan FV, Sorknaes AD, Tougaard L for the RYLUNG Group. Effect of diagnosis of "smoker's lung" [Letter]. *Lancet* 1997;**349**:253

5   Macfarlane JT, Holmes WF, Macfarlane RM. Reducing reconsultations for acute lower respiratory tract illness with an information leaflet: a randomised controlled trial in primary care. *Br J Gen Pract* 1997;**47**:719–22

6   O'Connor AM, Rostom A, Fiset V, *et al*. Decision aids for patients facing health treatment or screening decisions: systematic review. *BMJ* 1999;**319**:731–4

7   Grilli R, Freemantle N, Minozzi S, Domenighetti G, Finer D. Mass media interventions: effects on health services utilisation [Cochrane review]. In: *Cochrane Library*, Issue 3. Oxford: Update Software, 1999

8   Meredith C, Symonds P, Webster L, *et al*. Information needs of cancer patients in west Scotland: cross sectional survey of patients views. *BMJ* 1996;**313**:724–6

9   Wyatt JC, Keen JR. The NHS's new information strategy. *BMJ* 1998;**317**:900

10   Munro J, Nicholl J, O'Cathain A, Knowles E. Evaluation of NHS Direct first wave sites: second interim report to the DoH. Sheffield: Sheffield University Medical Care Research Unit, 2000

11   Pearson J, Dudley HAF. Bodily perception of surgical patients. *BMJ* 1982;**284**:1545–6

12   Wyatt JC. Measuring quality and impact of the World Wide Web. *BMJ* 1997;**314**:1879–81

13   Weisbord SD, Soule JB, Kimmel PL. Poison on line—acute renal failure caused by oil of wormwood purchased through the Internet. *N Engl J Med* 1997;**337**:825

14   Raynor DK, Yerassimou N. Medicines information—leaving blind people behind? *BMJ* 1997;**315**:268

15   Mayberry JF, Mayberry MK. Effective instructions for patients. *J R Coll Physicians Lond* 1996;**30**:205–8

16   Wyatt J. Evaluating electronic consumer health material. *BMJ* 2000;**320**:159–60

17   Wyatt JC, Wright P. Medical records 1: design should help use of patient data. *Lancet* 1998;**352**:1375–8

18   Graham W, Smith P, Kamal A, Fitzmaurice A, Smith N, Hamilton N. Randomised controlled trial comparing the effectiveness of touch screen system with leaflet for providing women with information on prenatal tests. *BMJ* 2000;**320**:155–60

19   Braddock CH, Edwards KA, Hasenburg NM, Laidley TL, Levinson W. Informed decision making in outpatient practice. *JAMA* 1999;**282**:2313–20

20   Borowitz S, Wyatt J. The origin, content and workload of electronic mail consultations. *JAMA* 1998;**280**:1321–4

6 Practice guidelines and other support for clinical innovation

Chapter 1 discussed how to formulate and pursue clinical questions. Looking up clinical questions during or immediately after patient care can be an effective method of learning: however, you must first realize your ignorance, then formulate a searchable question, find the answer and change your practice as a result. Even when there is widespread knowledge about an important innovation in clinical practice, such as aspirin for patients with myocardial infarction (MI), many patients are still incorrectly managed. Practice guidelines— 'systematically developed advisory statements created according to validated methodologies'[1]—act as a compact summary of the evidence and other factors guiding patient management so could be helpful in this context, but they are many and various[2,3].

How to select a guideline

Your consultant asks you to identify a guideline to increase the local use of aspirin after MI

As a perfectionist, you want to select the very best from the multitude of guidelines on management of MI. But what makes a good-quality guideline? Italian workers have proposed three criteria: whether the guideline (a) reports the range of professionals involved in development, (b) reports the strategy used to identify primary evidence and (c) explicitly grades the recommendations[2]. Inspection of 431 specialty society guidelines published from 1988 to 1998 showed that 54% met none of the criteria, 34% met one, 7% met two and only 5% met all three. Seemingly, speciality guidelines have been dominated by 'experts', with little involvement of GPs and other users. Equally, most guidelines result from an informal mélange of opinion in the charged social atmosphere of a committee. One encouraging result in the Italian review was that the more recent guidelines were more likely to include details of literature search and graded recommendations.

A UK group has developed a checklist of 37 questions exploring three dimensions (rigour of development, clarity of content and context, documentation of methods for application and monitoring) [www.sghms. ac.uk/phs/hceu/]. In a study in which six clinicians used this 'St

George's checklist' to assess 60 guidelines the inter-rater agreement was excellent[4]. However, even if a guideline is of high scientific quality, doctors may still not follow it. An observational study of Dutch clinicians suggested that key determinants of whether recommendations would be followed were that they were uncontroversial, specific, evidence-based and required no change to existing routine[5].

Even when we locate a satisfactory published guideline, it often proves too bulky or inconvenient for use in routine patient care. Some guideline authors now offer support tools such as glossy laminated flowcharts, pocket prompt cards or wall posters. Such tools are discussed later.

How to make a guideline locally relevant

Guidelines nearly always contain recommendations that cannot be universally adopted. For instance, certain tests or treatments may not be locally available, or a recommendation for specialist care may run counter, without supporting evidence, to a local tradition of community care. Thus, a national guideline commonly needs to be adapted if local clinicians are to get a feeling of 'ownership'. Strategies can include:

- Summarizing the guideline in a standard short format for a house officers' handbook
- Deleting the sections that do not apply locally (if there is no strong evidence that they should be retained)
- Adding information about local facilities and services, such as to whom to refer patients, which days the clinic takes place and what phone number to ring[6,7].

However, sometimes when scrutinizing and tailoring a guideline one realizes that the raw material is unsatisfactory and a new one is needed.

How to write a new guideline

After applying the St George's checklist to five guidelines on aspirin in MI, you find that none is satisfactory. You resign yourself to writing a definitive guideline Writing a high-quality guideline is hard, especially if you mean it to score well on the St George's checklist[4]. Before writing a single recommendation you will have to set up a multidisciplinary group, conduct detailed searches, appraise and grade the evidence, and combine this with other information such as patient preferences and health economic data. Various bodies, including the Scottish Inter-collegiate Guideline Network [www.sign.ac.uk][8]

and the North of England Group[9], have developed and published rigorous methods. Lessons from such activities are that adherence to the methodology depends not only on clinical commitment but also on library and epidemiological support, that the evidence tends to be more abundant than expected but much of it is of low quality, and that the effort of reaching agreement is about twice that envisaged. You decide to go ahead; but you are stopped in your tracks by your clinical director who asks about the legal implications for guideline users, authors and publishers.

What is the legal position of guideline users and authors?

Despite worries that the introduction of guidelines would lead to a flood of negligence cases, guidelines play a part in only 7% of US malpractice claims. However, there is a sufficient body of cases to allow some general conclusions[10,11].

Differences between clinical and legal views

Guidelines are created for a medical purpose, so have no special legal status. To a doctor, practice guidelines are clinical guidance resting firmly on the authority of science. To a lawyer, a guideline advises health professionals to practise in one way rather than another. Courts are always wary of guidance that cannot be subjected to cross-examination; so, although guidelines may be used in court to support a negligence case, they cannot substitute for expert testimony. An expert witness is necessary to help the court interpret the relevance of a guideline, even when its recommendations are found to be representative of responsible practice. Thus, the legal status of each guideline must be decided afresh in each case[10].

Liability of authors and publishers

As a matter of public policy and to encourage the dissemination of knowledge, book authors and publishers are 'never' found liable for negligence due to errors[12]. However, guidelines may be treated differently[10]. There have been no UK negligence cases yet, but in American courts the developers have been held liable for faulty guidelines. Commenting on the relevance of this to the UK, Hurwitz wrote: 'There appears to be no logical reason why similar liability could not attach to the originators and issuers of UK guidelines shown to cause patient harm as a result of faulty guideline development methods'[10]. Failure of the guideline user to protest about the guideline does not protect the developer from a claim of negligence. Even if patients generally fail in suing guideline authors, other parties (such as a company whose product is disadvantaged) may bring a case[11].

Guidelines are merely advice, so the language used should encourage and remind clinicians to exercise appropriate discretion, for example avoiding words such as 'never' and 'always'[10].

However, use of permissive language ('probably', 'sometimes') when directive terminology is more appropriate may not protect the developers from liability. Such permissive language would be troublesome if it encouraged users to assume that other actions were appropriate in circumstances when the evidence supported only one course of action.

Liability of doctors for adherence

Adherence to a guideline is not automatically evidence of reasonable clinical practice, so doctors cannot escape legal liability by claiming that adherence to a guideline has overridden their clinical judgment[10]. In the UK, even if a guideline has been agreed as a legal standard, appropriate application still requires discretion. For example, a Scottish man with congenital homonymous quadrantanopia successfully appealed for restoration of his driving licence even though it had been withdrawn on the basis of legally adopted guidelines. A clinician who complies without protest with an inappropriate guideline cannot then deny responsibility for patient harm. The test of reasonableness of medical treatment remains 'the standard of the ordinary skilled man exercising and professing to have that special skill... who acted in accordance with a practice accepted as proper by a reasonable body of medical men skilled in that particular art'[13].

Liability of doctors for non-adherence

In determining the status of a particular guideline, courts are likely to consider its authority, flexibility and scope, whether its development and application had statutory backing, and whether it embodies practices accepted as proper by a responsible body of doctors. Clinical practice may be perfectly lawful when it does not comply with a guideline, even one issued with executive authority. As Lord President Clyde stated in 1957, 'There is ample scope for genuine difference of opinion and one man is not negligent merely because his conclusion differs from that of other professional men'[10]. One reason for writing guidelines is to encapsulate recent innovations in clinical science. However, the existence of such a guideline does not make every clinician liable. Lord Denning stated in 1955 that 'It would be quite wrong to suggest a medical man is negligent because he does not at once put into operation the suggestion that some contributor or other might make in a medical journal'[10]. Guidelines designed to hasten the adoption of recent evidence would not reflect customary professional care.

Once your guideline group has taken these lessons to heart, it moves fast to produce a high-quality guideline which you succeed in publishing in a journal. The major question, now, is how to ensure that your guideline exerts the desired effects on clinical practice.

How to promote a clinical innovation

You spend a year developing a definitive guideline on aspirin and MI which you publish in a journal and also circulate locally. However, 6 months later local clinicians are still not advising patients to take aspirin after MI

Publication in a journal or circulation by mail is seldom sufficient[14,15]. Part of the challenge is to get clinicians to read the guideline, and strategies include filing a summary of the recommendations in patient notes, producing a summary card for clinic room desks or a wall poster, composing a page for the junior doctors' handbook, and making slides for continuing education. Techniques less specific to guidelines[16] include patient information leaflets, financial incentives and use of opinion leaders (Appendix 6.1 for definitions).

Before the innovator can select the appropriate technique or combination of techniques, he or she must understand the barriers to change. Some clinicians may need to be persuaded or actually helped to do what is recommended; moreover, waverers will require continuing encouragement if they are to persevere with the innovation in the face of counter-pressure from patients[17] or peers. These stages are summarized in the PRECEDE model[18]— predisposing people to innovation, enabling the innovation and reinforcing the innovation (Table 6.1).

Identification of barriers to innovation requires an understanding of where each individual or group lies in the innovation process and is fundamental to selection of appropriate techniques. Methods such as outreach visits[19] contain multiple elements effective against many barriers. As with broad-spectrum antibiotics we can say that they often work though we seldom know exactly why. Innovation techniques can be expensive and have serious unwanted effects. Again as with antibiotics, precise diagnosis beforehand will help in choice of a suitable agent. Table 6.1 links the three innovation stages, some specific barriers at each stage and appropriate techniques.

Effectiveness

A difficulty in determining the effectiveness of an innovation technique is the large number of variables. For example, the intended result may be to introduce a new procedure or to lessen use of an outmoded one. The clinical behaviour targeted may be ordering of laboratory tests (to aid diagnosis[20], screening or disease monitoring), prescribing, referral, hospital discharge or counselling[21]. A technique which works well in one of these areas may not be effective in another. Techniques may be used singly or in combination, and with or without an attempt to identify the barriers to innovation. A systematic review of 99 randomized trials, examining 160 innovation

Table 6.1 Barriers to clinical innovation and possible techniques to overcome them

Stage in the PRECEDE model	Documented barrier to innovation	Possible innovation techniques
1. Predispose to innovation (staff unwilling to change)	Clinicians do not know about it	Outreach visits; opinion leaders; wall charts; distance learning material; informal continuing education
	Apathy or lack of interest	Outreach visits; opinion leaders; incentives; audit of existing practice; provide information to patients; informal continuing education
	Concern about peer resistance	Target opinion leaders; informal continuing education; arrange focus group or survey of peers; provide distance learning materials
	Concern about patient resistance	Survey, involve and educate patients; social marketing techniques
	Conflicting financial interest	Remedy the perverse incentive: eliminate fees for obsolete services
	'We do it already'	Prospective self-audit (e.g. log book)
	'We're too busy'	Analyse, revise and agree job content; substitute staff; obtain more resources
	Too many innovations already in progress	Identify other staff to take the necessary action; prioritize and schedule innovations
2. Enable innovation (staff willing to change, 'system' is against them)	Poor access to high quality patient data	Case finding, care pathways, checklists for patients or clinicians; redesigned or computer-based records
	No access to detailed knowledge about innovation	Printed or computer-based guidelines or reference material; informal continuing education, opinion leaders, outreach visits
	Difficult to synthesize patient data with clinical knowledge	Informal role-playing seminars; case conferences; decision support systems
	Staff do not have the physical skills	Organize training courses; substitute staff who do have skills
	Staff do not have necessary space, staff, drugs, equipment	Identify and obtain the necessary resources
	'No money'	Reallocate funds from ineffective activities; seek increased budget (via managers, opinion leaders, patients, media)
	Medicolegal or risk management concerns	Seek clarification; involve patients, support groups, self-help groups
	Other organizational problems	Analyse and streamline care process (e.g. patient-focused care, re-engineering, quality improvement approaches)
3. Reinforce innovation (staff need continued encouragement)	Forgetting	Reminders; audit and feedback; staff rotation; refresher courses; incentives.
	Simple mistakes caused by action slips or capture errors	Redesign tasks to eliminate memorization Establish blame-free culture; log errors and near misses in an incident reporting system (Ref 22). Re-engineer care processes to make errors less likely, e.g. staff substitution, redesigned records and request forms

Table 6.2 Effectiveness of innovation techniques along four dimensions (data from Ref 16)

Dimension	Aspect	Effectiveness as per cent (No.) of techniques studied
Type of clinical behaviour targeted	Procedural skills	25% (1/4)
	Enhanced diagnosis	50% (2/4)
	General management of a problem (e.g. asthma)	55% (32/58)
	Resource utilization, including test ordering	71% (17/24)
	Preventive care activities	74% (40/54)
	Prescribing	79% (11/14)
Type of innovation technique studied	Formal continuing education course	14% (1/7)
	Educational materials	36% (4/11)
	Audit and feedback	42% (10/24)
	Patient mediated (e.g. leaflets)	78% (7/9)
	Reminders to clinicians	85% (22/26)
	Outreach visits	100% (7/7)
	Opinion leaders	100% (3/3)
Number of innovation techniques used	One innovation technique	60% (49/81)
	Two techniques	64% (25/39)
	Three or more techniques	79% (31/39)
Method used to identify barriers to innovation	No identification of barriers	42% (5/12)
	Literature showed need	53% (18/34)
	National guideline showed need	61% (25/41)
	Local consensus process	58% (26/45)
	A study to identify local barriers	89% (25/28)

techniques[16], indicated that 70% of techniques improved clinical practice and 48% improved patient outcomes. A rough idea of the effectiveness of these innovation methods along four dimensions can be had from Table 6.2, though the comparisons are almost never within a single study and the number of studies is often too small to provide a reliable estimate.

Other relevant material is included in Chapter 2 (continuing education) Chapter 5 (patient information) and Chapter 9 (decision support systems).

References

1   Field M, Lohr K, eds. *Guidelines for Clinical Practice: from Development to Use*. Washington DC: National Academy Press, 1990

2   Grilli R, Mgrini N, Penna A, Mura G, Liberati A. Practice guidelines developed by specialty societies: the need for critical appraisal. *Lancet* 2000;**355**:103–6

3   Hibble A, Kanka D, Pencheon D, Pooles F. Guidelines in general practice: the new tower of Babel? *BMJ* 1998;**317**:862–3

4   Cluzeau FA, Littlejohns P, Grimshaw JM, Feder G, Moran SH. Development and application of a generic methodology to assess the quality of clinical guidelines. *Int J Qual Health Care* 1999;**11**:21–6

5   Grol R, Dalhuisjsen J, Thomas S, in 't Veld C, Rutten G, Mokkink H. Attributes of clinical guidelines that influence use in general practice: observational study. *BMJ* 1998;**317**:858–61

6   Robins A, Gallagher A, Rossiter MA, Lloyd BW. Evaluation of joint medical and nursing notes with pre-printed prompts. *Qual Health Care* 1997;**6**:192–3

7   Riley K. Care pathways: paving the way. *Health Services J* March 26 1998:30–1

8   Miller J, Petrie J. Development of practice guidelines. *Lancet* 2000;**355**:82–3

9   Eccles M, Freemantle N, Mason J. North of England evidence based guidelines development project: methods of developing guidelines for efficient drug use in primary care. *BMJ* 1998;**316**:1232–5

10   Hurwitz B. Clinical guidelines and the law: advice, guidance or regulation? *Eval Clin Pract* 1995;**1**:49–60

11   Hurwitz B. Legal and political considerations of clinical guidelines. *BMJ* 1999;**318**:661–4

12   Brahams D, Wyatt J. Decision-aids and the law. *Lancet* 1989;**ii**:632–4

13   Bolam vs. Friern Hospital Management Committee. *All Engl Law Rep* 1957;**2**:118–22

14   Freemantle N, Harvey EL, Wolf F, Grimshaw JM, Grilli R, Bero LA. Printed educational materials: effects on professional practice and health care outcomes. In: *The Cochrane Library*, issue 3. Oxford: Update Software, 1999

15   Evans CE, Haynes RB, Birkett NJ, *et al.* Does a mailed continuing education package improve physician performance? Results of a randomized trial. *JAMA* 1986;**255**:501–4

16   Davis DA, Thomson MA, Oxman AD, Haynes RB. A systematic review of the effect of continuing medical education strategies. *JAMA* 1995;**274**:700–5

17   Macfarlane JT, Holmes W, Macfarlane R, Britten N. Influence of patients' expectations on antibiotic management of acute lower respiratory tract illness in general practice: questionnaire study. *BMJ* 1997;**315**:1211–14

18   Green LW, Eriksen MP, Schor EL. Preventive practices by physicians: behavioural determinants and potential interventions. *Am J Prev Med* 1988;**4**:101–7

19   Wyatt J, Paterson-Brown S, Johanson R, Altman DG, Bradburn M, Fisk N. Trial of outreach visits to enhance use of systematic reviews in 25 obstetric units. *BMJ* 1998;**317**:1041–6

20   Solomon DH, Hashimoto H, Daltroy L, Liang MH. Techniques to improve physicians' use of diagnostic tests. *JAMA* 1998;**280**:2020–7

21   Silagy C, Lancaster T, Gray S, Fowler G. The effectiveness of training health professionals to provide smoking cessation interventions: systematic review of randomised trials. *Qual Health Care* 1995;**3**:193–8

22   Brennan TA, Leape LL, Laird NM, *et al.* Incidence of adverse events and negligence in hospitalized patients. Results of the Harvard Medical Practice Study I. *N Engl J Med* 1991;**324**:370–6

23   Thompson O'Brien MA, Oxman AD, Davis DA, Haynes RB, Freemantle N, Harvey EL. Audit and feedback:

effects on professional practice and health care outcome. In: *The Cochrane Library*, issue 3. Oxford: Update Software, 1999

24   Adams ID, Chan M, Clifford PC, *et al.* Computer aided diagnosis of acute abdominal pain: a multicentre study. *BMJ* 1986;**293**:800–4

25   Wyatt JC. Clinical data systems, part II: Components and techniques. *Lancet* 1994;**344**:1609–14

26   Taylor P, Wyatt J. Decision support. In: Haines A, Donald A, eds. *Getting Research Findings into Practice*. London: BMJ Publishing 1998:86–98

27   Durand-Zaleski I, Rymer JC, Roudot-Thoraval F, Revuz J, Rosa J. Reducing unnecessary laboratory use with new test request form: example of tumour markers. *Lancet* 1993;**342**:150–3

28   Lomas J, Enkin M, Anderson GM, Hannah WJ, Vayda E, Singer J. Opinion leaders vs audit and feedback to implement practice guidelines. *JAMA* 1991;**265**:2202–7

29   Nutting PA, Beasley JW, Werner JJ. Practice-based research networks answer primary care questions. *JAMA* 1999;**281**:686–8

30   Chassin MR. Quality of health care part 3: Improving the quality of care. *N Engl J Med* 1996;**335**:1060–3

31   Wyatt JC, Wright P. Medical records 1: Design should help use of patient data. *Lancet* 1998;**352**:1375–8

32   Rowe R, Wyatt J, Grimshaw J, Gordon R. Manual paper reminders: effects on professional practice and patient outcomes (protocol for Cochrane Review). In: *The Cochrane Library*, issue 3. Oxford: Update Software, 1999

33   O'Connor AM, Rostom A, Fiset V, *et al.* Decision aids for patients facing health treatment or screening decisions: systematic review. *BMJ* 1999;**319**:731–4

34   Towle A, Godolphin W. Framework for teaching and learning informed shared decision making. *BMJ* 1999;**319**:766–71

35   Grilli R, Freemantle N, Minozzi S, Domenighetti G, Finer D. Mass media interventions: effects on health services utilisation. In: *The Cochrane Library*, issue 3. Oxford: Update Software, 1999

36   Wallace S, Wyatt J, Taylor P. Telemedicine in the NHS for the millennium and beyond. *Postgrad Med J* 1998;**74**:721–8

Appendix 5.1   Definitions of clinical innovation techniques

Audit and feedback	Collection and feedback of pooled activity or outcome data (Ref 23)
Business process re-engineering	Analysing the fundamental aims of an organization and how best to meet them
Care pathways	Preprinted multiprofessional record forms for common conditions or procedures, incorporating reminders (Refs 6,7)
Case conferences	Multidisciplinary discussion of specific cases and how to manage them
Case finding	Identification by staff or computer of patients who fulfil criteria for specific actions
Checklists for patients/clinicians	Proformas for patients or clinicians to prompt for data to be collected (Ref 24)
Computer-based records	Use of computers to enable flexible data collection and to search coded data (Ref 25)
Continuing education	Shared seminars, workshops, conferences, etc. The most effective allow participants to determine the agenda

Continuing professional development	Encouraging clinicians to recognize and address their training needs through whatever means are feasible and appropriate
Decision support systems	Computer systems which use patient data and clinical knowledge to generate patient-specific information or advice (Ref 26)
Distance learning material	Printed, video or computer-based material used to support learning which is posted or made available over the Web (Ref 14)
Incentives	Financial or other (e.g. peer group recognition)
Modified request forms	Redesign of paper or computer request forms to capture the information needed to support the innovation and eliminate inappropriate options (Ref 27)
Opinion leaders	Those professionals to whom others turn for advice; giving relevant information and distance learning materials to these individuals (Refs 23,25)
Outreach visits (synonym: counter-detailing)	A knowledgeable person visits clinicians, discusses the innovation, answers questions and leaves behind distance learning material (Refs 19,23)
Patient information	Providing preformed, tailored paper or computer-based information about a condition or procedure
Patient-focused care	Redesign of a clinical function to provide a one-stop shop for patients, incorporating all the resources required for routine patient management
Practice-based network	A primary care network to discuss and disseminate research methods and results (Ref 29)
Prospective self-audit	A variant of audit using self-collected data to ensure confidentiality and ownership of results
Quality improvement	Use of continuing quality improvement techniques, including audit, incident monitoring and definition of targets (Ref 30)
Record redesign	Redesign of paper or computer records to present critical patient data and other information in a suitable format to support the innovation (Ref 31)
Remedy perverse incentives	For example, reducing fees for unnecessary services (Ref 28)
Reminders to clinicians	Collection and feedback of patient data, clinical knowledge or advice relevant to individual patients by record inserts, stickers, stamps, etc. (Refs 16,32)
Reminders to patients	Reminder letters or phone calls to patients about their treatment, appointments, diet etc; may be combined with case finding, checklists, decision support systems (Ref 33)
Shared decision-making	Active involvement of patients and carers in choosing management options. Synonym: patient participation (Ref 34)
Social marketing	Survey, involve, provide information to and educate people in the community by health promotion techniques, advertising, telephone help lines, walk-in health shops, etc. (Ref 35)
Staff substitution	Substituting new staff, often more junior or more specialized, for some patient care activities
Telemedicine	Use of electronic media to communicate between patients and clinicians or between clinicians on more than one site (Ref 36)

SECTION 3
NEW TECHNOLOGIES AND THEIR CLINICAL ROLES

7 Intranets for knowledge access

An intranet is a private mini-Internet, cut off from the outside world (see Figure 7.1). Inside the intranet, people use linked computers to browse material held on the server or to send messages, files or other information in the same way as they use the Internet. If there is a special 'firewall' computer, authorized people on the intranet can also access material in the outside world on the Internet or NHSNet but no one in the outside world can access the organization's intranet (unless specifically permitted). The firewall acts like a one-way valve, so intranets are ideal for healthcare organizations, with their identifiable patient data and other confidential information[1].

Pros and cons

Why should a healthcare institution wish to install an intranet? First, organizations within the NHS have low budgets for information technology (IT), often relying on a range of out-of-date equipment and unable to insist that only one brand of personal computer (PC) is

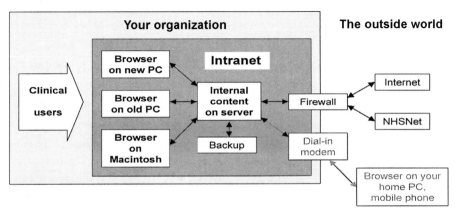

Figure 7.1   **How an intranet relates to your organization and the outside world**

Box 7.1 Benefits common to an intranet and the Internet

Everyone 'has' the latest version of every document: single organization-wide shared filing cabinet/library for documents and information with no duplication (unless it is copied or printed out)

Anyone can join in: browsers work on every platform and most operating systems, even obsolete Macs, PCs, Suns or personal data assistants

Easy navigation: browser programs provides 'back' and 'forward' buttons and easy access to a list of recently browsed pages

Fast complete detailed searches: all documents are held in electronic form and indexed

Easy customization: users can readily 'bookmark' a document or page by adding it to their list of favourites in the browser

Easy sharing of expensive hardware such as high-capacity file server, high-volume printers, automatic-feed optical mark readers (for patient surveys or research)

Eases training and support: web browsers are a single universal program; 'thin clients' and 'application sharing' mean that the same software package is installed once by an expert and downloaded to your computer

Allows access to multimedia: e.g. for training and reference

Allows access to masses of data: web servers can construct pages dynamically from information held in databases.

---

installed. Because free or inexpensive e-mail and web browsing software are available for nearly every kind of computer, including obsolete PCs and Macintoshes, an intranet is an ideal low-cost way to link these up and allow users of heterogeneous systems to access material throughout the organization.

Second, once employees are familiar with browsing the organization's intranet from one computer, they will be able to perform the same and other tasks from any linked computer. With the limited NHS budget for IT training opportunities, this is useful.

Third, the speed of change in healthcare means that the chosen computing system must be very flexible and capable of development with minimum input from expensive IT staff[1]. Intranets satisfy this requirement well, even allowing information from numerous 'legacy' systems to be brought together on one screen[2]. The other implication of rapid change is that NHS organizations create and revise mountains of paper documents (general practitioners receive 15 kg of guidelines alone every year[3]). An intranet means that only one copy of each document—the current version—is maintained and available, and any authorized person who needs to refer to it can do so, from any linked machine. Because the document is held on a central server with daily backup, it is safer than one held on the author's office PC. To ensure that no document copies—paper or electronic—are needed, every person who needs access should be granted it, whenever and wherever he or she works. A consultant holding an outreach clinic at a health centre or working from home will need to use documents or data

Table 7.1 Benefits of a local intranet over the Internet

Local intranet	Unrestricted access to Internet
Allows a sense of ownership: provides a first stop before the Internet, with local news and information	No local ownership: content of the first stop before the Internet depends on the particular Internet service provider used
Directs staff to local high-quality content relevant to the organization, with no distractions	Hugely varying content, many distractions
Maintaining confidentiality of local material is simple: firewall automatically isolates intranet from outside world	Maintaining confidentiality is complex: requires knowledge, administration of passwords, etc.
Organization oversees intranet content, architecture and security, how staff access the wider Internet	Organization has less control over content, how staff access the Internet
Differential access: access levels can be tailored to different professional groups, roles, functions, etc.	No differential access
Allows quality improvement: the organization can measure use of intranet resources to improve its information services	Hard to implement quality improvement, e.g. monitor staff use of remote sites, provide guidance, improve quality of content
Allows economical access to licensed material: bulk site licence for material cheaper than many individual licences; well-designed intranet ensures that licensing conditions will not be violated	Expensive *ad hoc* access to licensed material: more expensive; staff may share passwords etc., violating licensing conditions
Improved performance and reliability: organization can invest in local network and servers to improve performance	Variable speed and reliability: at the whim of the Internet services provider; often limited to 56k modem link

held on the trust intranet. This means extending the trust network beyond obvious physical boundaries—for example, by using a secure dial-in route as shown in Figure 7.1. Careful configuration is needed to ensure this does not become a back door for unauthorized access; one approach is a 'defender' system, which receives your call then dials you back on a previously authorized number. Access to intranets from third-generation mobile phones will also be needed soon, since these devices may replace phones, pagers and PCs for many staff who never even leave the building during office hours. In future, we may move toward larger closed health intranets, to support continuity of care and mobile health workers in community care organizations[4] or bigger health regions[5].

Fourth, finding a paper document—especially the latest version—can be a headache, even when you know exactly which document you want. It is much harder when all you know is that a document must exist somewhere on the topic. An intranet is like an electronic library, holding all documents in digital form with a detailed index; thus you can search by text words or key words, even when you do not know where it is or what it is called. Box 7.1 summarizes the general benefits of both an intranet and the Internet, while Table 7.1 contrasts specific benefits of an intranet with those of a direct link to the Internet.

Drawbacks

On the minus side, setting up an intranet is not always technically or organizationally straightforward. It can be expensive, with costs including:

- Capital costs of the server and firewall and of installing a high-capacity network with ubiquitous access points
- Revenue costs of staff to support and maintain the network and intranet server, to train users and contributors
- Costs of obtaining material, whether externally licensed or internal. For example, licensing of a few bibliographic databases and a score of full-text journals to an NHS hospital intranet might cost around £10 000 a year. Costs also include the time spent by staff on assembling, organizing and updating internally contributed material.

Some of this expenditure may be necessary for other purposes, such as electronic prescribing or picture archiving systems.

What other drawbacks? Here are a few. The organization is responsible for any abuse of copyright material—for example, if people scan textbook images onto their pages. By preventing staff from accessing the Internet in an *ad-hoc* way, the organization takes on the responsibility of training users to get best out of the intranet; some users may resent restriction of their access to the Internet because the firewall prevents them downloading programs or setting up an open-access Internet server. Once connected to an intranet, an internal rogue user or virus has greater access to other people's information. A single linked machine which also has a modem connection to the Internet can also threaten the security of the whole intranet. Finally, where a partner organization already has its own intranet, there is sometimes a dilemma about whether to join it or build your own. Failure to address this in one UK teaching hospital gave rise to three network points on the wall behind every PC in the oncology unit—one each for the NHS Trust, the medical school and a major cancer charity.

An understanding of the distinctions between an intranet and the Internet and the potential drawbacks of intranets is only the first step in exploiting this attractive technology. One further possibility, allowing the user the benefits of access to the Internet as well as the intranet, is to extend the intranet outside the organization to a few carefully selected Internet sites, such as Royal Colleges or providers of licensed content. This approach has been called the extranet model.

Clinical applications of intranets

Publishing and browsing static content

This is the traditional application of intranets, to enable clinicians and others to access a variety of documents, including:

- Browsing 'frequently asked questions' with clear, concise, answers on topics of importance to the organization
- A local bulletin board, perhaps with the current issues of local newsletters and an archive of past issues
- Lists of current research in progress, courses and conferences, etc.
- Documents about quality standards and performance; the organization's annual report, listing how each department matched up to these standards
- Junior doctors' or laboratory handbooks, local policy documents
- The local formulary and book of local or national practice guidelines.

Accessing databases over an intranet

Clinicians will be familiar with use of computers in a library to access knowledge sources such as drug information (WeBNF [www.pharmpress.rpsgb.org.uk], Micromedex), Clinical Evidence [www.clinicalevidence.org], electronic textbooks, bibliographic tools, library catalogues and full-text journals (e.g. Ovid [www.ovid.com]). However, such knowledge sources can be networked over an intranet to give access from your desktop PC. In a recent French study, this doubled the use of Medline, leading to many more searches relevant to patient care[6]. The same technology can allow access, via a web browser, to information traditionally held in rather hostile databases. Such data might include:

- Patient data—a master patient index with patient demographics or more clinical information such as laboratory, radiology or endoscopy[7] reports or even a full electronic patient record[2] or picture archiving and communications system[8]
- A directory of local people, services and clinics, held in frequently updated form in a database
- A directory of all drugs available, with their characteristics[9].

Interactive tasks

Increasingly, clinicians are using communications and information technology to assist in more complex tasks. In the past this often meant learning the quirky commands of specific software tools, but many of these functions can now be achieved through a web browser operating over an intranet. Here are some examples:

- Communication: sending and receiving e-mail to individuals or discussion lists, both internal and external to the organization. When combined with on-call schedules, a calendar and work schedule, a personnel directory and a clinical information system, this can greatly improve departmental function[10]
- Decision support tools ranging from a simple form with blanks to calculate anion gap or risk of ischaemic heart disease to a complex computer model such as the Heart Disease Program[1]
- Interactive learning resources such as patient simulators or complex case data combined with multi-choice questions. Many institutions already have much material that can be converted to intranet format[11], or it can be written from scratch. For example, in Sydney, 400 faculty members have placed material on their intranet to support the new problem-based undergraduate medical curriculum[12]
- Booking of NHS resources, such as outpatient appointments or meeting rooms; ordering reprints from a library; scheduling a meeting with peers by use of their web diary
- Collaboration tools such as a shared departmental reference database or tools for joint authoring, submission and tracking of a research project
- Telemedicine tools for referral and case discussion by use of 'lean' videoconferencing or store-and-forward techniques[13,14]. Linkage of neurosurgical stereotactic instruments to an intranet has even been reported[15].

New applications of intranet techniques are constantly being invented; see the Oxford clinical web applications directory [www.oxmedinfo.jr2.ox.ac.uk/cwap/dir.taf?fhome]. The NHS Plan[16] makes extensive reference to the use of such technology to improve clinical practice and patient outcomes, but so far few if any of the above have demonstrated such benefits in rigorous studies.

Commissioner perspective

From the perspective of the organization, an intranet needs high-level support and this can be part of the strategy for quality, human resources, risk or knowledge management. Construction and maintenance of an intranet, and training people about it, is an ideal role for library and information services staff, who are already experts in indexing, PC training, networking, Internet and intranet technology, and negotiating access to copyright material. It is *not* a project that can be left to the IT department. This is because a well designed intranet needs to:

- Include high-quality information: content should be regularly checked for accuracy and currency by those who provide it
- Be easy to browse: logical organization, consistent design
- Be easy to search: across the whole site, similar documents, within a single document
- Be comprehensive: provide access to most of the resources that staff need most of the time, allowing access to relevant external Internet sites
- Be fast and reliable: minimum network or server delays, up-time 99.5% or more, few dead links
- Preserve confidentiality: appropriate use of password controls
- Provide added value over the Internet / own resources: linking related information (e.g. a drug formulary with electronic prescribing system, evidence-based information about laboratory tests to a laboratory report[17])
- Reinforce local identity: include information of interest to the organization—news, organization chart, who's who, functions, resources.

To build and maintain an intranet that meets all of these criteria is hard, but the task can be eased by software tools such as server log analysers and web spiders which automatically map and check links, index pages and check page download times. Getting the first version up and running is greatly helped by saving word-processor files in the HTML format used by web browsers or as PDF files for viewing by use of Adobe Acrobat. However, in the long run the material will need to be formatted specifically for the intranet medium, moving away from simple linear documents. Many of the tasks required cannot be automated, and individuals contributing material must adhere to a loose style guide, otherwise every page or section on the intranet will look different and users will become disoriented. It is also important to devise a comprehensive logical menu structure for the whole site, content being fitted in as it becomes available, and to identify and apply a controlled vocabulary of index terms. Every page must be dated and the webmaster needs tools for linking pages to authors and revision dates. There are various useful sources of design principles for intranet-based electronic health records[1,2,18].

Conclusions

With all the superlatives about the Internet, organizations may be slow to realize that equal or greater benefits are available to them from installing an intranet. Intranets have most of the advantages of Internet technology and very few of the disadvantages. However, developing a successful intranet does require investment and a strategic view. At present it is hard to say whether an intranet is the key factor in those few NHS organizations that have achieved 'modernization', or whether their intranet is merely a marker of organizations with a clear sense of purpose.

References

1   Fraser HSF, Kohane IS, Long WJ. Using the technology of the world wide web to manage clinical information. *BMJ* 1997;**314**:1600–3

2   McDonald CJ, Overhage JM, Dexter PR, *et al*. Canopy computing: using the Web in clinical computing. *JAMA* 1998;**280**:1325–9

3   Hibble A, Kanka D, Pencheon D, Pooles F. Guidelines in general practice: the new tower of Babel? *BMJ* 1998;**317**:862–63

4   Reddy S, Niewiadomska-Bugaj M, Reddy YV, *et al*. Experiences with ARTEMIS—an internet based telemedicine system. *Proc AMIA Annu Fall Symp* 1997:759–63

5   Shortliffe EH. The evolution of electronic medical records. *Acad Med* 1999;**74**:414–19

6   Darmoni SJ, Benichou J, Thirion D, Hellot MF, Fuss J. A study comparing centralised CD-ROM and decentralised intranet access to MEDLINE. *Bull Med Libr Assoc* 2000;**88**:152–6

7   Sackmann M, Rosette R, Busl T, *et al*. A scientific relational database combined with a report generator for endoscopy in networks: EndoNet. *Endoscopy* 1998;**30**:610–16

8   Gropper A, Doyle S, Dreyer K. Enterprise scale image distribution with a Web PACS. *J Digit Imaging* 1998;**11**(suppl 1):12–17

9   Francois M, Joubert M, Fieschi D, Fieschi M. Implementation of a database on drugs into a university hospital intranet. *Medinfo* 1998;**9**(part 1):156–60

10   Willing SJ, Berland LL. A radiology department intranet: development and applications. *Radiographics* 1999;**19**:169–82

11   Dugas M, Batschkus MM, Lyon HC. Mr Lewis on the web—how to convert learning resources for intranet technology. *Med Educ* 1999;**33**:42–6

12   Carlile S, Barnet S, Sefton A, Uther J. Medical problem based learning supported by intranet technology: a natural student centred approach. *Int J Med Inf* 1998;**50**:225–33

13   Wallace S, Wyatt J, Taylor P. Telemedicine in the NHS for the millennium and beyond. *Postgrad Med J* 1998;**74**:721–8

14   D'Souza M, Shah D, Misch K, Ostlere L. Dermatology opinions via intranet could reduce waiting times [Letter]. *BMJ* 1999;**318**:737

15   Oizumi T, Ohira T, Kawase T. The use of computers and networking in the neurosurgical field. *Rinsho Byori* 1999;**47**:119–25

16   Milburn A. *The NHS Plan: a Plan for Investment, a Plan for Reform*. London: Stationery Office, 2000

17   Kay JD, Nurse D. Construction of a virtual EPR and automated contextual linkage to multiple sources of support information on the Oxford clinical intranet. *Proc AMIA Annu Fall Symp* 1999:829–33

18   Smith RA, Arvanitis TN, English M, Vincent R. An intranet database for pacemaker patients. *Int J Med Inf* 1997;**47**:79–82

8 The Internet and clinical knowledge

With its variety, promises and even vices, the Internet resembles the physical world. This chapter will not describe every way clinicians or patients can use the Internet; Robert Kiley's *JRSM* series and book[1] are a good resource. Instead it discusses use of the Internet to find and assess knowledge, to answer clinical questions and to assist lifelong learning. Other chapters discuss the formulation of clinical questions (Chapter 1), lifelong learning in general (Chapter 2), use of the medical literature (Chapter 3), helping patients with Internet print-outs (Chapter 5) and characteristics shared with Intranets (Chapter 7).

The Internet is a worldwide network consisting of many smaller networks, all using the same protocol to exchange messages. Many computer tools exploit this protocol, including electronic mail, file transfer protocol to download files, and the worldwide web.

Electronic mail as a clinical tool

Though apparently dull in comparison with the web, electronic mail is a key Internet application for person-to-person communication, even allowing telemedicine by attachment of digital photographs or video clips to messages. Use of e-mail for patient-to-doctor communication is increasing[2], and can be useful in the opposite direction. There are many medical discussion lists focusing on specific topics—see [www.mailbase.ac.uk/other/medi-class.html] for a directory. A well-chosen discussion list is the perfect place to float a burning topic or publicize a conference, and can be a useful way to get answers to clinical questions. However, the time to response and quality of the answers are very variable. The 'frequently asked questions' section list archive can provide a short cut, if the question has been satisfactorily answered.

The worldwide web

The web consists of a linked network of websites and of pages within them. A page can contain anything from text, data entry forms or pictures to video, sound, a computer program or even virtual reality simulation. Simple 'browser' tools help us navigate the web by following links and store bookmarks to pages we might want to find again. Static web pages are generated from word-processed documents or written with a simple mark-up language called HTML. Dynamic pages are generated on demand by a program—for example, a database report or customized list. There are now a hundred million websites and billions of web pages. Websites come in three main kinds (Table 8.1).

- Sites providing content (text, pictures, etc., arranged as a book or newsletter)
- Sites providing services (e.g. patient-specific advice generated by a human or computer program, a sales catalogue/ordering service; data collection forms for a survey)
- Search tools to help you find the right website and pages within it, resembling 'Yellow Pages' (directory site) or a book index (search engine).

Increasingly, providers are tailoring content to the user, offering services, while new 'portal' sites bring together a rich mixture of content and services under one virtual roof. However, you should remember that many portal and directory sites receive a commission for linking to certain sites.

Getting directly to the information you need

With this profusion of web content and services, it is easy to forget that information is only useful if it is relevant to your problem, valid and easy to find and access. Slawson expressed this neatly in a formula[3]: usefulness=relevance × validity/work to access.

A huge variety of search tools (e.g. [www.yahoo.com], [www.google.com]) will help you find material on the web. There are search sites which submit your query to a dozen other search engines (e.g. [www.metacrawler.com]) and some will interpret your free-text question and find the answer for you (e.g. [www.askjeeves.com]). There are also medicine-specific search engines. Hardin MD ([www.lib.uiowa.edu/hardin/md]) offers a comprehensive list of other sites with useful lists of medical sites. In a recent study of 10 common primary care questions[4], nine medicine-specific search engines answered an average of only one question while Hardin MD, Excite and HotBot (general search engines) each answered five and a content provider, MD Consult ([www.mdconsult.com]) answered six.

Table 8.1 Characteristics of the main types of websites

	Content provider	Service provider	Search tool	Web portal
Examples	National electronic library for health	Internet bookshop; helps doctors and patients find a doctor with specific skills		Single site offering comprehensive links to content and services; help user find sites matching stated criteria
Main role	Originate content	Provide interactive service	Direct user to any site based on search string	
Coverage	Narrow—a single specialty, topic	Medium—often several topics	Everything from annuities to Zaire	Narrow–wide
Assemble content	Yes	Maybe	No	Maybe
Quality assure content	Maybe	Maybe	Maybe	Yes
Links to relevant sites	Maybe	Maybe	Yes	Yes
Browsing method	Page of links; may include on-site search tool	Page of links	On-site search tool	Pages of links; may include on-site search tool
On-site search tool	Maybe	Maybe	Always	Maybe
Include/consult experts in topic	Maybe	Often	Maybe	Maybe
Bias possible	Yes	Yes	Yes	Yes
Commercial	Maybe	Often	Often	Often
User pays to access	Maybe	Often	No	Maybe

Marshall[5] provides sound advice on searching the web with 10 frequently used search engines. To summarize, if you want whole sites devoted to a distinct subject, use a directory tool such as Yahoo or About ([www.about.com]). If you are looking for a specific piece of information, use a conventional search engine such as AltaVista ([www.altavista.co.uk]). However, these match on all sites containing your search word, so, enter as many words as you can and use the 'advanced search' options to narrow the choice. Use lower case, unless it is a specific phrase, which should be in quote marks ("Great Ormond Street"). Some engines even allow you to search only for image or sound files (to use in slide presentations, for example). For non-medical searches, Ask Jeeves turned out to be the fastest and most complete in a simple test.

Looking for high quality information

Finding a long list of sites that contain the phrase you searched for is easy, but assuring relevance and validity is much harder. Because the web allows anyone to publish anything, they do. A casual search for sites about cancer or back pain will turn up thousands, with alarming claims based on commercial bias or simple naivety[6]. These assertions are sometimes read and acted on by web users, with serious results[7]. One good strategy is to stick with recognizable brand names—of journals, societies or professional organizations with a reputation to lose. However, this means missing the thousands of high quality sites assembled by enthusiastic amateurs, the same people who could never afford to publish via traditional media.

One way round this difficulty is to take advantage of website owners who are careful about the sites to which they link. Sites with many links to them—which form the core 30% of websites[8] (Figure 8.1)—tend to be reliable and up-to-date (which is why other sites link to them). The number of links to a page can serve as a surrogate for its validity and relevance. The Google search engine ranks sites matching a simple Boolean search by the number of links to them, and is a recommended fast route to reliable material in the web core or origination sites.

An alternative to such technical criteria is for a human being to visit every website and check whether it passes basic thresholds for relevance and validity—for example, does it state the author, the source of material and the date of publication[9]. The Open Directory project uses human indexers ([www.dmoz.org]) and supplies results to search engines including AltaVista, which includes a detailed catalogue of approved sites. Medical indexers using clinical criteria construct the medical catalogues at OMNI ([www.omni.ac.uk]) and Medical Matrix ([www.medicalmatrix.com]). Clearly no single project can cover more than a tiny fraction of the web, and keeping the index up to date is a challenge. One possibility might be worldwide collaboration, perhaps using a technique called PICS labels[10]. A more modest approach to finding linked, reliable sites uses web rings. A web ring consists of sites about a topic linked together so that users can navigate forward or backward, or to a random linked site. Some web rings have no selection criteria but most refuse to allow biased or unreliable sites to join. Thus, for minority interests such as patients' experiences with a rare disease, a web ring may be useful. A directory of web rings is on [www.webring.org].

An alternative to employing an army of independent reviewers is to publish a code of practice, and allow website owners to place your badge on their site if they fulfil your code. The Health on the Net Foundation ([www.hon.ch]) was one of the first to do this and many health sites now carry its badge. However, some sites do not actually fit HON criteria, broad though they are. Finally Quackwatch ([www.quackwatch.com]) includes a list of bizarre and speculative therapies on offer on the web, and advice about how to avoid them.

Other troubles with the Internet

Limited access to the Internet in National Health Service organizations is a continuing difficulty. In a survey of Yorkshire general practitioners only half had any access to the Internet, and less than a quarter had easy access, often at home[11]. A survey of NHS librarians in 1999[12] uncovered a wide range of excuses given by NHS trusts for failing to provide them with Internet access, casting doubt on the NHS progress in improving knowledge management.

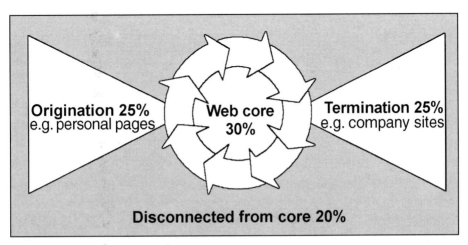

Figure 8.1 **The 'bow tie' structure of the web** [adapted from Ref 8]

In surveys, three-quarters of members of the public using health websites are concerned about privacy. Whereas medical librarians have a clear ethical code there are currently no ethical obligations on websites, or even non-medical web health services, to protect privacy. 'Leaky' browser software and advertising banners can capture personal information even without you knowing it, and one web advertising company has been sued as a result. There is also sometimes a mismatch between a site's declared privacy policy and what is actually done (see [http://ihealthcoalition.org] for a Hudson survey report). Remedies include the e-Health ethical code (see later), disabling the cookie function on your browser, checking the privacy policy of any site before you fill out forms and using [www.anonymizer.com] as an intermediary when surfing.

Some other negative aspects of health and the Internet are listed in Table 8.2.

Using the Internet to support clinical tasks

Answering clinical questions

In theory, by providing rapid access to clinical knowledge the Internet could assist clinical consultations. Librarians using conventional Medline searches alone were able to answer one-third of 84 clinical questions to the satisfaction of family physicians[13], but this took 27 minutes compared with 6 minutes using a medical textbook. However, although faster, the textbook answered only one-sixth of the questions. Web access to Medline is easy ([www.ncbi.nlm.nih.gov/entrez/query.fcgi]) but answering questions still takes time and skill and the conclusions of primary studies and informal reviews are hard to find and unreliable[14].

Using a primary care branch of the National Electronic Library for health ([www.nelh.nhs.uk]), I was able to obtain evidence-based summary answers to a handful of clinical questions from Cochrane review abstracts or Bandolier in about 40 seconds—quite promising, though this still means a minute or two not communicating with my patients. Other evidence tools which contain a short 'bottom line' and may be useful include the CAT bank ([www.jr2.ox.ac.uk/cebm]), Clinical Evidence ([www.clinicalevidence.org], registration required) and Bandolier itself ([www.jr2.ox.ac.uk/bandolier]). Evidence-based guidelines can be found at [www.sign.ac.uk]. Speciality sites also exist; for example [www.rcsed.ac.uk.uk/fmi/gateway.asp] is an excellent page of surgical and other links. An on-line dermatology atlas could help GP decision making, but full-screen diagnostic images can take minutes to download—[www.derma.med.uni-erlangen.de/bilcldb/index_e.htm].

Table 8.2 Some negative aspects of the Internet and e-health

Problem	Possible solutions
Loss of personal contact/therapeutic relationship	Individual e-mail responses; telephone response to patient e-mails
Inaccurate, biased information	Codes of conduct; filtering, labelling, portals
Easier suicide because of wider access to how-to guides	Codes of conduct; balanced discussion of issues
Economic failure of conventional journals and book publishers	Migrate to Internet/hybrid publishing
Munchausen by Internet—people pretending to have serious conditions	Awareness
More rapid spread of bogus cures, misinformation, e.g. about laetrile	Codes of conduct
Unfounded campaigns against individual clinicians and institutions	Clarify rules of libel
Tidal wave of information—not surfing but drowning	Personalized newsletters, search tools
Erroneous policies based on naïve web surfing	Education of public and policy makers—*caveat lector*
Exaggerating the gap between the information rich and poor	Provide Internet access in public libraries, other languages, take account of sensory defects; provide Internet learning resources—[www.netskills.ac.uk]

There have been few systematic studies of the accuracy and completeness of web searches to answer clinical questions. Hersh[15] observed practising physicians to capture 50 questions such as 'do anabolic steroids cause gallstones?' To answer each, a medical librarian used Metacrawler to interrogate multiple Internet search engines. This retrieved a total of 629 pages (mean 13 pages, range 2–20 per question). Only 11% of these pages were directly applicable to the query and there was at least one applicable page for 26 (52%) of the questions. Only 40% of pages were oriented to professionals and 58% of pages were reviews but only three (0.5%) were systematic reviews. Turning to basic quality criteria, the authors were indicated in 31% of pages, a source in 12%, the site affiliation was clear in 53% and the date of writing in 18%. Potential conflicts of interest and financial support were indicated in 12%.

In their comparison of different methods for finding material, Graber *et al.*[4] concluded that generic search engines were much more useful than medical ones but that the Hardin MD service and MD Consult ([www.mdconsult.com]) answered the most questions and passed the most quality criteria.

Using the Internet to support education and learning

Although the Internet is barely yet able to support decision making during patient care, it does offer a wide range of content and services to support learning. With 400 000 new papers added to Medline annually, there is a desperate need for current awareness services. WebMedLit ([www.webmedlit.com]) scans many medical websites daily—including most major medical journals—and e-mails free specialty-specific newsletters. Other update services include UpToDate ([www.uptodate.com]), Infotrieve for Medline ([www.infotrieve.com]), Northern Light ([www.northernlight.com]) for new web pages and Amazon for new medical books[16]. Some individual content providers offer an update service including the *BMJ*'s weekly e-mailed contents ([www.bmj.com]) or the monthly FDA MedWatch drug safety newsletter ([www.fda.gov/medwatch/safety.htm]).

If you see an article you need, check if it is in one of 200 medical journals available free on the Internet at [www.freemedicaljournals.com]. If not, services such as Infotrieve's Docsource allow you to browse 22 000 journal titles, find what each article costs and how long it will take, and order the ones you want. However, charges for some document supply services are high.

There are a wide range of other commercial content providers on the web including MDConsult, UpToDate and Ovid ([www.ovid.com]). For $35 per month clinicians can subscribe to MDConsult, which allows access to over 120 titles including 40 reference and textbooks, 30 journals, most of the *Clinics of North America* and 45 Yearbook titles. UpToDate is edited by former editors of the *Annals of Internal Medicine* and forms an official part of the US Society of General Internal Medicine's educational activities. It is sponsored by several major specialty societies and contains a comprehensive range of material synthesized from many sources, including 130 journals scanned monthly. It is available as a CD-Rom updated 4-monthly for those with a poor Internet link. Like Clinical Evidence it is question focused and includes reviews written by over 1800 experts. It was used more frequently than MDConsult, Medline or Scientific American Medicine Online in a recent University of Alberta study. Ovid provide a wide range of bibliographic databases, the full Cochrane Library and Best Evidence content, full text journal articles and 35 books as well as Clinical Evidence as part of its product range, but is usually subscribed to by medical libraries or organizations rather than individuals. An innovative Australian project, the Clinical Information Access Project ([www.clininfo.health.nsw.gov.au]) offers a comprehensive range of such resources to over 80 000 clinicians in four states. Some of the major medical portals such as WebMD ([www.webmd.com]) include access to similar content in their subscription rates.

Assessment is part of any learning programme. The web offers a variety of ready-made multiple-choice questions and even tools to prepare one yourself, needing no knowledge of HTML ([www.dmoz.org/Computers/Software/Marketing/Surveys]). High-fidelity patient simulations serve a similar purpose. As early as June 1996[17], Diabetes UK placed a diabetes simulator on its site to help patients and professionals explore the impact of insulin and diet on 24-hour glucose profile. Biomednet ([www.biomednet.com], registration required) offers various free resources to support learning and research including a medical webzine and 'evaluated Medline containing expert-selected, annotated articles'. Usefully, Biomednet remembers your personal search history for later. There are also tools such as an interactive anatomy tutor for FRCS candidates ([www.vesalius.com]) and interactive grand rounds ([www.cyberounds.com]) offering CME credits by e-mail and experts to answer your questions in private or in public. Respected organizations such as the European School of Oncology have set up excellent educational websites ([www.cancerworld.org]). Although these are often sponsored by the pharmaceutical industry, an independent advisory board should help assure quality and independence of content.

One drawback of the web is slow download times. Delays are mostly due to local links, not the Internet backbone[18], and can be completely overcome by publishing material with the same web mark-up and browser technology on a CD. An example is a CD version of *Robbins Pathological Basis of Disease* containing 17 chapters and 1000 pathological images on one CD[19]. However, keeping such resources up to date is a serious challenge.

With this plethora of web learning resources, we should ask how the web compares with, say, a definitive textbook that has evolved over multiple editions. Lim *et al.*[20] selected a past anaesthesia fellowship exam paper randomly then sought information to answer each of the 15 questions using the textbook index to look up key words and synonyms from questions. Textbook information was judged adequate to answer nine (60%) questions, inadequate for two and absent in four. The median time taken to retrieve the answer was 25 minutes (range 10–55). AltaVista was then used to search the Internet with the same words and spelling variants. This provided an answer to every question within the first 50 hits for each search; all but two answers were judged adequate. In total 38 sites were used and there were no contradictions between facts on the Internet and the textbooks. However, searching the Internet took a median of 110 minutes (range 60–150)—at least four times as long. Thus, although the Internet provided a wider range of information than a single textbook, it was much slower to search—adding over 21 hours to answer all 15 questions.

Thus, given time and a knowledgeable searcher, the Internet can provide a wider range of answers than print sources. Access to the Internet resources does allow learners, course developers and tutors to be separated in space and time, and can be complemented by a

Box 8.1 Summary of the e-health code of ethics

Candour	Sites should clearly state the owner and purpose of the site, and describe the relationships between content providers and others
Honesty	Sites should be honest in all content and claims about products and services, distinguishing adverts from content
Quality	Sites should provide accurate, well supported information, products and services; use best evidence and qualified practitioners for personal advice; indicate the origin of information (opinion, studies ...); editorial policy for educational/research sites; add the date of publication, of revision and the sources used to each page; include a statement of how the site evaluates content and links to other sites
Informed consent	Sites should obtain affirmative consent for the collection and use of personal health information; state what data are collected, for whom, how they are used, who they are shared with and the consequences of refusal
Privacy	Sites should take reasonable steps to protect personal information; make it easy for users to review any personal information held on them and trace how this information is actually used; say how information is used and for how long it is stored; ensure that deidentified data cannot be linked back to individuals
Professionalism	On-line health providers should: abide by professional ethics (do no harm, put patient's interests first, protect confidences, disclose conflicts of interest, state fees, obey local laws); state their identity, location and qualifications; describe the terms and conditions of the interaction; try to understand client's circumstances and identify their local health resources; give clear follow-up information; inform patients about the constraints of online activity; help e-patients understand when to use online and when to use face to face consultations
Responsible partnering	Sites should: make reasonable efforts to ensure that partners and sponsors abide by the law and uphold the same ethical standards; insist that sponsors do not influence the way search results are displayed; indicate whether links are for information only or indicate endorsement of those sites; indicate when users are leaving the site
Accountability	Sites should: indicate to users how to contact the site owner or manager; provide feedback tools; review complaints promptly, responding in appropriate ways; encourage users to notify them if partners, affiliates or linked sites violate legal or ethical principles; monitor their own compliance with the code of ethics

web-based learning log allowing you to update it from wherever you are[21]. This permits students to work flexibly when and where they choose, even from home or in another country, and may help integrate basic sciences and clinical disciplines[21].

Using the net to support clinical innovation and quality improvement

Clinical innovation (Chapter 6) and quality improvement include setting objectives, assessing current performance, determining reasons for imperfect performance and deciding how to move toward the objective. Internet resources can clearly help with setting objectives, and are useful also at other stages of the process. For example, one early study described how the Internet can be used to share and exchange cytopathology images for diagnoses across a national external quality assurance scheme[22], reducing transcription errors, administrative costs and delays. E-mail discussion lists may also help by allowing those attempting to bring about change to share their knowledge and experience.

Conclusions

Despite their drawbacks, e-mail and the web do offer us numerous sources of information and services to help working doctors manage their knowledge. Location of relevant information is time-consuming, and few resources are yet speedy enough for use during clinical consultations. However, the web is already widely used for continuing learning and is an excellent vehicle for this. As John Chambers, chief executive of Cisco Systems (who make the hardware the Internet runs on), said: 'Education over the Internet is so big it's going to make e-mail look like a rounding error'. But none of this will take off until the average web user can identify reliable unbiased material. One recent proposal which may help is the e-Health code of ethics ([www.ihealthcoalition.org]) which covers all sites providing health information, products and services (see Box 8.1). How many sites will take this new code to heart remains to be seen.

References

1   Kiley R. *The Doctor's Internet Handbook*. London: RSM Press, 2000

2   Borowitz S, Wyatt J. The origin, content and workload of electronic mail consultations. *JAMA* 1998;**280**:1321–4

3   Slawson DC, Shaughnessy AF, Bennet JH. Becoming a medical information master: feeling good about not knowing everything. *J Family Practice* 1994;**38**:505–13

4   Graber MA, Bergus GR, York C. Using the World Wide Web to answer clinical questions: how efficient are different methods of information retrieval? *J Family Practice* 1999;**48**:520–4

5   Marshall G. Fetch! Net magazine April 2000 issue 69 ([www. netmag.co.uk/print.asp?id=20494])

6   Jadad AR, Gagliardi A. Rating health information on the Internet. Navigating to knowledge or to Babel? *JAMA* 1998;**279**:611–14

7   Weisbord SD, Soule JB, Kimmel PL. Brief report: poison on line—acute renal failure caused by oil of wormwood purchased through the Internet. *N Engl J Med* 1997;**337**:825

8   Sherman C. New Web map reveals previously unseen "bow tie" organizational structure [www.infotoday.com/newsbreaks/nb000522-1.htm]

9   Wyatt JC. Measuring quality and impact of the World Wide Web [commentary]. *BMJ* 1997;**314**:1979–81

10   Eysenbach G, Diepgen TL. Towards quality management of medical information on the Internet: evaluation, labelling, and filtering of information. *BMJ* 1998;**317**:1496–502

11   Anon. *Access to the Evidence Base From General Practice in Northern & Yorkshire Region.* York: NHS Centre for Reviews & Dissemination, 2000

12   Carnnall D. NHS librarians cannot access the Internet. *BMJ* 1999;**319**:10

13   Chambliss ML, Conley J. Answering clinical questions. *J Family Practice* 1996;**43**:140–4

14   Antman EM, Lau J, Kupelnick B, Mosteller F, Chalmers TC. A comparison of results of meta-analyses of randomized control trials and recommendations of clinical experts. *JAMA* 1992;**268**:240–8

15   Hersh WR, Gorman PN, Sacherek LS. Applicability and quality of information for answering clinical questions on the Web [Letter]. *JAMA* 1998;**280**:1307–8

16   Kiley R. Current awareness services on the Internet. *He@lth Info Internet* 2000;No. 15:1–2

17   Lehmann ED. Diabetes moves on the Internet. *Lancet* 1996;**347**:1542

18   Wood FB, Cid VH, Siegel ER. Evaluating Internet end-to-end performance: overview of test methodology and results. *J Am Med Inform Assoc* 1998;**5**:528–45

19   Carlson JA. Digital interactive pathogenesis [Review]. *Lancet* 1999; **354**:1309

20   Lim MJAJ, Ho KM. A comparison of the Internet and a standard textbook in preparing for the professional anesthetic examination. *J Clin Monit* 1999;**15**:449–53

21   Neame R, Murphy B, Stitt F, Rake M. Universities without walls: evolving paradigms in medical education. *BMJ* 1999;**319**:1296–300

22   Rashbass J, Vawer A. A networked computer program for managing a national external quality assurance scheme in cytopathology. *Cytopathology* 1996;**7**:377–85

9 Clinical decision support systems

A clinical decision support system (DSS) is a computer program that provides reminders, advice or interpretation specific to a given patient at a particular time[1]. These systems differ from bibliographic or other search tools in their use of patient data to drive a 'reasoner' program that searches a knowledge base to assemble a tailored report. The differences are summarized in Table 9.1.

Kinds of clinical decision support system

Some DSSs are designed for use by the public—for example, a web-based cardiac risk calculator ([www.allhealth.com/sponsors/zocor/calculator.html]). Those for health professionals include an anticoagulant dosage calculator[2], an AIDS reminder system[3], and the tools used by NHS Direct nurses to triage 12 million cases per annum[4].

DSSs can also be embedded in medical instruments such as electrocardiographs[5] or lung function recorders[6]. Others are integrated into general-practice or hospital information systems, and these can issue not only routine reminders but also urgent alerts about test orders, laboratory results or possible drug interactions[3]. In one study such a system led to more rational test ordering and reduced inpatient length of stay by a day—though at the cost of requiring junior doctors to spend 6 minutes extra per patient per day ordering tests[7].

Do we need decision support systems?

A first question is, do clinicians *want* decision support? A survey of 403 Internet-literate UK doctors (41% general practitioners), all members of the Medix Internet service provider, showed that in 1 month 60% would use a Royal College guideline, 55% a flowchart and 39% a checklist but only 24% would use a computer-based decision support system; 33% would never use one. Are these doctors right to judge DSSs less acceptable than guidelines, flowcharts or checklists? One drawback of guidelines and flowcharts is their proliferation[8],

Table 9.1 Factors distinguishing decision support systems from bibliographic and other search tools

	Decision support systems	Search tools
Use	System automatically assembles context specific advice or reminder using patient data	User formulates a search string; system retrieves potentially relevant text; user sorts through results to find relevant material
Input	Patient data, suitably coded, often obtained direct from electronic patient record	Text search string and/or coded search terms entered by human user
Output	Dynamically constructed reminder or advice	A list of performed text chunks (e.g. abstracts) matching the search string
Knowledge base	Machine-readable facts, assembled by a knowledge engineer or clinician using a knowledge editor	Human-readable prose and coded index terms selected by librarians, entered by clerks
Smallest knowledge unit	Discrete medical fact (e.g. a drug indication)	Text 'chunk', a sentence to a whole chapter in length (e.g. an abstract)
Search process	Reasoner program uses patient data to search knowledge base with predefined algorithms	Boolean search program matches search string against text or index terms, ranks results using a relevance score
Scope	Usually narrow—e.g. a single problem or disease	Wide—e.g. the journals covering one discipline

while another is difficulty tracing the path of a patient at a given encounter, even if you have the right guideline. Van Wijk used a randomized trial to compare the ability of a computer-based standard 15-item checklist and a DSS-generated problem-specific list derived from national guidelines to reduce the number of tests ordered by 66 Dutch general practitioners[9]. For those GPs randomized to the standard list there was a 12% reduction in the number of tests per order form, but the reduction was 29% (2.4 times greater) with the problem-specific DSS. Overall, the DSS led to 20% fewer tests ordered per GP than the standard checklist. Thus, despite the reluctance of computer-literate doctors to use DSSs, these systems can be more effective than their preferred tools such as a paper or computer based checklist.

An alternative analysis requires understanding of how DSSs might overcome barriers to clinical innovation (Chapter 6). The PRECEDE model[10] suggests that, to innovate, we must first predispose doctors to change by informing them of the innovation, then enable them to change by providing the necessary resources, and finally reinforce the change. A wide range of techniques including DSSs are available to assist this process, but should only be applied after consideration of the personal and organizational barriers to change. Some barriers that

Table 9.2 How decision support systems (DSSs) can overcome barriers at each stage in the clinical innovation process

Stage (Ref 10)	Barrier to innovation	Possible benefit from decision support system
1. Predispose to innovation (staff unwilling to change)	Clinicians do not know about innovation	Might help when used as a learning tool
	Apathy	Installation might attract clinical interest and generate discussion
	Peer resistance	DSS might help in marketing
	Patient resistance	DSS might promote innovation to patients
	'We're too busy'	DSS could empower nurse practitioner to take on the new task, freeing medical time
	Conflicting financial interest	Unlikely to help
2. Enable innovation (staff willing, 'system' is against them)	Patient data not complete, poorly presented	DSS issues problem-specific checklist or reminder to record relevant data, preinterprets complex patient data, carries out automatic case finding
	Poor access to detailed knowledge	DSS as intelligent front end to literature, filtering knowledge according to current patient and problem
	Clinicians find it hard to synthesize patient data and knowledge	DSS carries out complex calculation or logical reasoning to link relevant patient data and clinical knowledge
	Lack of skills	DSS might help when used as a learning or simulation tool
	Lack of space, drugs, equipment, money; medicolegal or other organizational problems	Unlikely to help
3. Reinforce innovation (staff need encouragement)	Forgetting	Reminders for clinicians (and patients)
	Mistakes caused by action slips, capture errors	Reminders and alerts to build a safe operating environment; preinterpreted patient data; problem-specific work-flow and record formats to lessen errors
	Diminished motivation over time	Reminders or alerts; DSS can help support others (e.g. nurse practitioners) to carry out routine tasks

can occur at each of the three innovation stages are listed in Table 9.2, with suggestions about how decision support systems might help overcome most of them: clearly, DSSs have the potential to assist at all three innovation stages, particularly when they are used to educate patients and clinicians, to support staff substitution or to enhance data capture and interpretation.

This leads on to the question, when do DSSs actually change clinicians' decisions, actions and patient outcomes?

When do decision support systems work?

Friedman *et al.*[11] examined the influence of two commercial diagnostic DSSs on the decisions of 216 US doctors confronted with difficult case scenarios[11]. Overall, the correct diagnosis appeared on 40% of doctors' differential diagnosis lists pre-DSS and 45% post-DSS—an 11% increase in diagnostic accuracy. In 12% of cases, the DSS caused doctors to put the correct diagnosis on their list but in 6% it caused them to drop the correct diagnosis, giving a net gain of 6%. The net gain was largest for students (9%) and smallest for faculty (3%). The QMR system[12] produced a net gain of 8%, twice that of the ILIAD system (4.1%). Thus a DSS, if it is to improve performance substantially, needs to be well designed and to be used by relatively inexperienced doctors. On some occasions a DSS causes doctors to override their own correct decisions.

How often DSSs improve clinical decisions is less important than how often they lead to more appropriate actions and patient outcomes[1,13]. Hunt[14] systematically reviewed 68 randomized trials of DSSs from 1974 to 1997. Improvement was seen in 43 (66%) of the 65 trials with an endpoint of clinical performance and six (43%) of the 14 with an endpoint of patient outcome. Most interesting was the way in which the percentage of studies showing improvement varied according to the behaviour targeted:

- Diagnosis: one (20%) of five studies
- Drug dosing: nine (60%) of 15 studies
- Active clinical care: 19 (73%) of 26 studies
- Preventive care: 14 (74%) of 19 studies.

This shows that the typical complex diagnostic DSS is rarely effective—perhaps because routine clinical practice poses few diagnostic challenges, because doctors already excel at diagnosis or because doctors pay little attention to what emerges from such systems. However, the simple reminder systems that advise on active or preventive care frequently do lead to improved actions. Despite many years of development, complex diagnostic systems currently seem a solution looking for a problem.

A further question is, how do DSSs compare with other innovation methods? Davis *et al.* reviewed 101 randomized trials of innovation methods, again checking how many led to improved clinical practice, with the following results[15]:

- Formal continuing education course: 1/7 (14%)
- Educational materials: 4/11 (36%)
- Audit and feedback: 10/24 (42%)
- Patient mediated (e.g. leaflets): 7/9 (78%)
- Reminders to clinicians (e.g. DSS): 22/26 (85%)
- Outreach visits: 7/7 (100%)
- Opinion leaders: 3/3 (100%)

This showed that simple reminder systems were more effective at improving clinical actions than continuing medical education, audit and feedback, mailed educational materials or patient-mediated interventions, but less effective than the typical methods used by the pharmaceutical industry. One concern about these results is that they came from a wide range of settings, so perhaps the DSSs were used on clinical practices that were easier to alter. The only rigorous way to determine whether DSSs are more effective than another innovation method is to conduct a comparison within a single study. However, there are very few within-study comparisons. I have already mentioned one showing that DSSs were more effective than a standard checklist for containing test orders[9]. In another trial, a DSS was compared with a DSS combined with a team intervention, for improvement of drug ordering[16]. The expensive team intervention brought no additional benefit.

One factor that will obviously influence the acceptability of a DSS, and also its effectiveness, is the source of its knowledge[17].

Source of knowledge for a decision support system

All too often in the past the knowledge for DSSs has been acquired by a computer scientist or a knowledge engineer from a single expert—or even by browsing out-of-date narrative textbooks, with all their defects[18]. A handful of systems such as QMR[12] were constructed after informal literature reviews, while Preop was the first in which the knowledge engineering team used a critical appraisal process and tagged each fact in the knowledge base with its level of evidence[19]. A more recent example of a DSS based on reliable evidence is an ischaemic heart disease risk adviser used daily at a London teaching hospital[20]. The knowledge on which all advice is based derives from regression equations fitting the Framingham dataset.

With the growth of secondary literature such as Cochrane reviews and *Clinical Evidence*, it is now much easier for those building DSSs to assemble the knowledge base direct from relevant evidence. However, whether you are building a DSS or writing a practice guideline, the goal is to give advice rather than simply précis evidence. As well as the relevant evidence, therefore, makers of DSSs need to include information on such matters as preferences, policies and resource availability. If an evidence-based guideline already exists which has assimilated all this information, this makes the perfect starting-point for a DSS knowledge base (Figure 9.1).

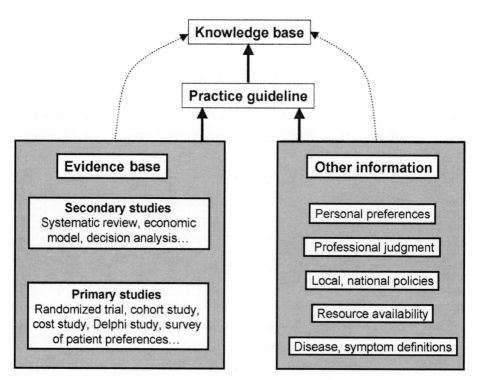

Figure 9.1   The roles of evidence and other information in practice guidelines and decision support systems

Box 9.1 Some criteria for a clinically useful decision support system (adapted from Refs 17 and 26)

The knowledge is based on the best evidence available (e.g. an evidence-based practice guideline or risk score)

The knowledge covers the problem in sufficient breadth and depth to allow sophisticated problem solving, advice and explanations

To ensure flexibility, the knowledge can be readily updated by a clinician without unexpected effects

To promote lifelong learning, the knowledge base links to related local and Internet material (images, practice guidelines...)

To make the system easy to use, most patient data are drawn from existing electronic sources

The performance of the entire system is validated against a suitable gold standard (Ref 27)

The system improves clinical practice or patient outcomes in a rigorous study (Refs 1, 25)

The clinician is always in control, so can receive advice, browse the knowledge base, get help and explanations, try out 'what-if' scenarios and obtain a critique of the patient management plan

The system is easy to access—for example via the world wide web [e.g. the Heart Failure Program (Ref 28) or an infective endocarditis advisor for developing countries (Ref 29)]

Conclusions

DSSs are a seductive technology with the potential to lessen information overload and reduce clinical oversights. However, we should remember that there will often be more than one way to resolve a problem—medication errors, for example[21]. Although DSSs can help at each of the three main innovation stages, it would be wrong to conclude that they are always the correct solution[22].

One reason to think twice before developing or buying a DSS is that these systems do have important drawbacks. As with many information systems[23], there is a risk that an expensive, inflexible DSS will freeze an organization's policies and procedures at one historical moment. DSSs can also be unpredictable[24], needing rigorous evaluation[1,25] to ensure that they are indeed improving clinical practice. Few DSSs will be used unless most of the patient information can be drawn from other routine data sources in suitably coded form. This means that they require substantial infrastructure, in the form of networks, electronic patient records and ubiquitous terminals (which need to be used frequently if clinicians are to receive alerts and reminders promptly). For example, in the Safran study of outpatient reminders[3], the median time till doctors responded to a computer-generated alert was 11 days: the reason for this delay was they did not use the computer regularly. Box 9.1 lists some criteria for a clinically useful DSS.

DSSs also raise complex professional and medicolegal issues. For example, to avoid exposure to liability, every DSS must treat its user as a 'learned intermediary'[30]. Consequently, black-box reasoners such as neural networks are clinically dubious[31]. Lately, a GP was sued after prescribing antacids for an epilepsy patient; the antacids had precipitated a seizure, causing the patient's driving licence to be withdrawn. The GP had inferred that, because there had been no alert from his prescribing system, no hazard would arise. However, although the system 'knew' that antacids are contraindicated in epilepsy and that the patient was receiving phenytoin, it did not 'know' that phenytoin is an antiepileptic drug. It was thus unable to deduce that the patient had epilepsy and that antacids were contraindicated.

Currently, although DSSs work well in certain clinical niches, their overall cost-effectiveness compared with other innovation methods is unclear. It also remains to be seen whether the complex systems developed with advanced 'artificial intelligence' functions have greater impact, or are easier to maintain, than the simple reminder and algorithm systems already widely used in electronic patient records and for nurse triage.

References

1   Wyatt J, Spiegelhalter D. Field trials of medical decision-aids: potential problems and solutions. In: Clayton P, ed. *Proceedings of 15th Symposium on Computer Applications in Medical Care, Washington DC, 1991*. New York: McGraw Hill, 1991:3–7

2   Poller L, Shiach CR, MacCullum PK, *et al*. Multicentre randomised study of computerised anticoagulant dosage. European Concerted Action on Anticoagulation. *Lancet* 1998;**352**:1505–9

3   Safran C, Rind DM, Davis RB, *et al*. Guidelines for management of HIV infection with computer-based patient's record. *Lancet* 1995;**346**:341–6

4   Munro J, Nicholl J, O'Cathain A, Knowles E. Impact of NHS Direct on demand for immediate care: observational study. *BMJ* 2000;**321**:150–3

5   Willems JL, Abreu-Lima C, Arnaud P, *et al*. The diagnostic performance of computer programs for the interpretation of electrocardiograms. *N Engl J Med* 1991;**325**:1767–73

6   Wyatt J, Denison D. ILTARS: an expert system to interpret the results of pulmonary function tests [Abstract]. *Thorax* 1989;**44**:327

7   Tierney WM, Miller ME, Overhage JM, McDonald CJ. Physician order writing on microcomputer workstations. *JAMA* 1993;**269**:379–83

8   Hibble A, Kanka D, Pencheon D, Pooles F. Guidelines in general practice: the new tower of Babel? *BMJ* 1998;**317**:862–3

9   Van Wijk MAM. BloodLink: computer based decision support for blood test ordering. Assessment of the effect on physicians' test ordering behaviour. [PhD thesis]. Rotterdam: Erasmus University, 2000

10 Green LW, Eriksen MP, Schor EL. Preventive practices by physicians: behavioural determinants and potential interventions. *Am J Prev Med* 1988;**4**(suppl 4):101–7

11 Friedman CP, Elstein AS, Wolf FM, *et al*. Enhancements of clinicians' diagnostic reasoning by computer based consultation. *JAMA* 1999;**282**:1851–6

12 Miller R, Pople H, Myers J. INTERNIST-1: an experimental computer-based diagnostic consultant for general internal medicine. *N Engl J Med* 1982;**307**:468–76

13 Heathfield HA, Wyatt J. Philosophies for the design and development of clinical decision-support systems. *Meth Inform Med* 1993;**32**:1–8

14   Hunt DL, Haynes RB, Hanna SE, Smith K. Effects of computer-based clinical decision support systems on physician performance and patient outcomes: a systematic review. *JAMA* 1998;**280**:1339–46

15   Davis DA, Thomson MA, Oxman AD, Haynes RB. A systematic review of the effect of continuing medical education strategies. *JAMA* 1995;**274**:700–5

16   Bates DW, Leape LL, Cullen DJ, *et al*. Effect of computerised physician order entry and a team intervention on prevention of serious medication errors. *JAMA* 1998;**280**:1311–16

17   Wyatt JC. Use of medical knowledge systems: lessons from computerised ECG interpreters. In: Barahona P, Christensen J, eds. *Knowledge and Decisions in Health Telematics*. Amsterdam: IOS Press, 1994:73–80

18   Antman EM, Lau J, Kupelnick B, Mosteller F, Chalmers TC. A comparison of results of meta-analyses of randomized control trials and recommendations of clinical experts. *JAMA* 1992;**268**:240–8

19   Holbrooke A, Langton K, Haynes RB, Mathieu A, Cowan S. PREOP: development of an evidence-based expert system to assist with preoperative assessments. In: Clayton P, ed. *Proceedings of 15th Symposium on Computer Applications in Medical Care, Washington DC, 1991*. New York: McGraw Hill, 1991:669–73

20   Hingorani AD, Vallance P. A simple computer program for guiding management of cardiovascular risk factors and prescribing. *BMJ* 1999;**318**:101–5

21   Bates DW. Using information technology to reduce rates of medication errors in hospitals. *BMJ* 2000;**32**:788–91

22   Delaney BC, Fitzmaurice DA, Riaz A, Hobbs FDR. Can computerised decision support systems deliver improved quality in primary care? *BMJ* 1999;**319**:1281–3

23   Keen J, Wyatt J. Back to basics on NHS networking. *BMJ* 2000;**321**:875–8

24   Fox J, Das S. *Safe and Sound: Artificial Intelligence in Hazardous Applications*. London: AAAI/MIT Press, 2000

25   Randolph AD, Haynes RB, Wyatt JC, Cook DJ, Guyatt GH. Users' guides to the medical literature: XVIII. How to use an article evaluating the clinical impact of a computer-based clinical decision support system. *JAMA* 1999;**282**:67–74

26   Wyatt J. Computer-based knowledge systems. *Lancet* 1991;**338**:1431–6

27   Wyatt JC, Altman DG. Prognostic models: clinically useful, or quickly forgotten? *BMJ* 1995;**311**:1539–41

28   Fraser HSF, Kohane IS, Long WJ. Using the technology of the world wide web to manage clinical information. *BMJ* 1997;**314**:1600–3

29   Karlsson D, Ekdahl C, Wigertz O, Shahsavar N, Gill H, Forsum U. Extended telemedical consultation using Arden syntax based decision support, hypertext and WWW technique. *Methods Information Med* 1997;**36**:108–14

30   Brahams D, Wyatt J. Decision-aids and the law. *Lancet* 1989;**ii**;632–4

31   Wyatt J. Nervous about artificial neural networks? *Lancet* 1995;**346**:1175–7

10 Conclusion: managing explicit and tacit knowledge in health services

Knowledge can be classified broadly as either explicit or tacit[1]. Explicit knowledge consists of facts, rules, relationships and policies that can be faithfully codified in paper or electronic form and shared without need for discussion. By contrast, tacit knowledge (or intuition) defies recording. This kind of knowledge underlies personal skill, and its transfer requires face-to-face contact or even apprenticeship.

Over time, some tacit knowledge does become amenable to analysis and decomposition, allowing recording in explicit form. An example is the evidence-based interpretation of diagnostic tests, in which the emphasis is on prior probabilities and likelihood ratios[2] rather than intuitive judgment. But we still hear the argument that by making tacit knowledge explicit we destroy it, or that most knowledge exists in the work of effective teams—'knowledge in action'[3]. I disagree: much of the medical progress in modern times has been attributable to an evolution from tacit to explicit knowledge, and its sharing with other groups including patients and the public.

In a key paper Hansen *et al.*[4] match the two kinds of knowledge to two kinds of problem, two kinds of professional and two knowledge-management strategies. The strategies are codification and personalization. Codification means identifying, capturing, indexing and making available explicit knowledge to professionals who are team players, willing and able to apply the knowledge in solution of everyday problems. Personalization means providing creative problem solvers—individuals with the tacit knowledge to solve one-off problems—with the means to identify and communicate effectively with other experts. The distinctions between and implications of these two strategies are explored in Table 10.1.

Knowledge management strategies for health services

One of the challenges of healthcare is that routine questions and tasks are intermingled with one-off, ill-formed, strategic dilemmas. This means that both strategies for knowledge management are needed, in ratios that will differ between functional units. Thus a unit that

Table 10.1 Comparison of strategies to manage explicit and tacit knowledge, based on Hansen (Ref 4)

	Codification for explicit knowledge (people to documents)	Personalization for tacit knowledge (people to people)
Intended result for organization	Uniform, high quality solutions to most problems; contain current risks and costs	Unique, appropriate, creative solutions to strategic problems; exploit opportunities and contain future costs and risks
Type of problem targeted and solution preferred	Routine, short-term, low-risk problem for which a good-enough solution is available but is not usually applied	One-off, medium to long-term, high-risk, strategic problem with no precedent needing a novel, customized solution
Knowledge management goal	Re-use of explicit knowledge by capturing, codifying, classifying and making available knowledge to support routine problem solving	Sharing of tacit knowledge by helping staff to identify relevant experts and enhance conversations to create novel solutions
Lego analogy	Re-using Lego bricks to build a range of models	Creating a new Lego product, e.g. Mindstorms control system
Type of professionals targeted	Implementers: bright graduate team players, trained in groups, willing to apply methods developed by others	Highly paid inventors: creative analytical thinkers trained one to one by mentors
Primary user questions	What problem is this, how does the organization usually respond?	What form might a solution take, who might know about this?
Typical knowledge management tools and techniques used	Library of procedure and policy documents, guidelines, data collection forms, typical cases, risk assessment tools accessible from all parts of the organization	Online CV, list of skills and publications for staff and external experts; e-mail discussion lists; regular case meetings, workshops and road shows; video-conferencing; co-locate staff, provide coffee area, staff secondments
Source of the knowledge being managed	Professional analysts working to the organization's agenda	Creative experts, whether internal or external, working to the problem owner's agenda
Level of IT and knowledge management investment	Intensive investment, justified by multiple knowledge re-use	Modest investment, justified by improved frequency and quality of communications
Staff incentives to encourage system use	Reward the use of and contributions to document databases; recognize staff adherence to policies	Reward direct communication with or being contacted by others; recognize experts and original solutions
Typical commercial organization	Service industry, provider of customized goods	Strategic consultancy, research, e.g. Hewlett Packard product development team
Matching NHS organizations	NHS Direct, primary care, PCG, health authority, NHS trust, NHS Supplies	Tertiary care centre, NHS Executive, NHS Estates

82

deals largely with routine cases might wish to expend 80% of its knowledge management resources on the codification strategy, while a unit in which most patients require creative solutions might devote 80% to the personalization strategy. By definition, routine patient management problems occur most frequently in front-line clinical units such as NHS Direct and general practice, and in district hospitals services that deal with a chronic disease affecting a single body system, such as asthma, ischaemic heart disease or epilepsy.

Examples of knowledge codification strategies adopted by the NHS for routine problem areas include the National Service Frameworks, guidelines from the National Institute for Clinical Excellence (NICE), care pathways and the triage algorithms used in the NHS Direct Clinical Advice System. The aim is to disseminate a standard approach based on best NHS practice, to move toward uniform reliable patient management and support systems and to raise performance to that of the best units. Such an approach should also help to simplify the organization of services, reduce anomalies such as postcode prescribing, reduce errors, contain costs and simplify clinical governance.

However, the NHS still has a long way to go to achieve the goal of providing ready access to and regular use of codified knowledge to solve most common problems. One reason is that many clinicians are highly educated analytical thinkers with an individual streak, reluctant to share their own knowledge or to apply codified knowledge developed by others in the cause of greater uniformity and better organizational performance. This is not our fault: at school and university we were rewarded for keeping our knowledge to ourselves and taught that to copy others was cheating[5]. As doctors we tend to look for differences between patients and for rare problems rather than applying well-worn solutions. We still select medical students from high academic achievers and train doctors to invent solutions by teaching them basic sciences and encouraging them to do research. We also use one-to-one clinical mentoring even though staff more readily apply uniform strategies for routine problems when they are trained in multiprofessional teams[4]. We certainly do not yet have a library of policies and procedures, standard data collection forms or risk assessment tools accessible from all parts of the organization, even if we have recently employed a handful of clinicians working to the organization's agenda to develop these (see Table 10.1).

A further obstacle arises from our failure to invest in the technology and infrastructure required by the codification strategy. High-quality knowledge must be available quickly enough to be useful. Compare what happens in business. Ernst and Young's Centre for Business Knowledge employs 250 well-qualified professionals, with a further 40 in each practice area (equivalent to a clinical specialty) to identify, capture, codify and disseminate good practice from company documents[4]. The NHS, with 20 times as many professional staff and a much greater problem throughput, can boast five professional staff in the National Electronic Library for Health together with two dozen employed by NICE and the National Service Framework authoring process.

Limits of the codification strategy

It is not only clinical care that sometimes demands a creative approach and exchange of tacit knowledge. Creative problem-solving is also needed to advance healthcare development, which Sir Michael Peckham defines as the process in which 'innovative use is made of knowledge and information to turn ideas and technologies into the provision of better, affordable health care'[6]. We do have modest informal networks and other methods for tapping the intuition of clinical and strategy experts in the NHS, industry, medical schools and elsewhere, but much more could be done, with the techniques suggested in Table 10.1, to implement this personalization strategy. However, most problems—whether in patient care, health promotion, service delivery or performance management—are by definition routine, and acceptable solutions can usually be assembled from existing evidence[7], guidelines or expert consensus. What is more, since routine problems occur frequently, a learning organization can enhance its codified knowledge by monitoring adverse outcomes and investing in quality improvement[8].

An alternative view of healthcare is that every patient and encounter is unique, so that each poses the clinician with a different dilemma requiring a creative individual solution. However, it is unwise and impractical for every clinician to indulge in creative problem solving for every patient—or even a substantial minority. If every management plan has to be created from the ground up, with all its uncertainties, this risks reinvention, ignores existing knowledge, and abdicates our professional responsibility to manage patients according to what society can afford. Treating common problems with widely agreed and carefully validated solutions is also faster and less likely to introduce error, misunderstanding and inequalities, and should be more efficient. This is not the same as saying that the NHS should offer only one therapy for each disease. It could follow the example of the personal computer manufacturer Dell, which applies a knowledge codification strategy in order to offer its customers 40 000 validated alternative products[9].

Management of tacit knowledge

Previous chapters have discussed evidence for the effectiveness of techniques for managing codified knowledge such as practice guidelines (Chapter 6), decision support systems (Chapter 9), tools for empowering patient choice (Chapter 5), access to reference databases

(Chapter 3) and the Internet (Chapter 8). However, few research groups have explored techniques for managing tacit knowledge in healthcare. Einbinder *et al.*[9] targeted referrals, developing a map of the process of selecting consultants and populating this with patient and provider preferences, to assist better informed choice based on a wider range of criteria. O'Brien *et al.*[10] expended much effort simply obtaining up-to-date information about consultant specialties and other services from NHS organizations. They then incorporated these data into a comprehensive electronic directory, which they provided to 19 GPs. The GPs who used the directory rated it easy to use and fast to learn from and preferred it to paper-based information for use during consultations. Evidence that members of a clinical specialty do exchange and accumulate tacit knowledge comes from a systematic review of studies examining knowledge, practices and practice outcomes of cardiologists and others[11]. Cardiologists were more knowledgeable than other clinicians about the investigation and management of ischaemic heart disease but not, surprisingly, about the use of angiotensin converting enzyme inhibitors for heart failure. Patients with ischaemic heart disease or heart failure were more likely to receive evidence-based care and have good outcomes when managed by cardiologists than when managed by generalists. The advantage of specialist care has also been shown for asthma patients managed by UK chest physicians[12].

Conclusions

The future of knowledge management in health is bright. We already have adequate technology in the shape of the Internet and a good intellectual framework in evidence-based health, which are being used to improve each other[13]. We also have many health librarians who are knowledge management professionals[14]. Computer tools for helping health professionals manage explicit knowledge, developed in the 1980s, have been greatly refined[15].

Recognizing that knowledge and knowledge workers are the key asset of any health system, the NHS has already started a programme of knowledge codification to inform routine problem solving. This includes developing a National Electronic Library of Health and appointing a senior library policy maker as a regional director of knowledge management and research and development. However, more needs to be done[16], including clarifying the two strategies described above, and linking these strategies with those for human resources, clinical governance, quality improvement, risk management and patient participation. Knowledge is every professional's concern, so the best policy may be to appoint specialty knowledge advisers or champions, rather than a chief knowledge officer in every NHS trust[17]. An economic analysis indicates that, when specialties and health organizations collaborate and share explicit knowledge in this way, each gains more than it invests[18].

Turning to tacit knowledge, we do already have some informal networks and a few tools to assist in the identification of and communication with experts. The personalization strategy for knowledge management does need to be developed, but not at the expense of distracting clinicians, policy makers and funders from the key task of making agreed explicit knowledge readily available in suitable forms. Finally, a key lesson from industry is that knowledge management programmes must not be confined to departments such as human resources or information technology but linked closely with strategic decisions made by senior professionals and policy makers[5]. Let me close with what Matheson[14] said in 1995:

'The overarching informatics grand challenge facing society is the creation of knowledge management systems that can acquire, conserve, organise, retrieve, display and distribute what is known today in a manner that informs and educates, facilitates the discovery of new knowledge and contributes to the health and welfare of the planet.'

References

1   Miller P. *Mobilising the Power of What You Know*. London: Random House, 1998

2   Jaeschke R, Guyatt GH, Sackett DL. Users' guides to the medical literature III. How to use an article about a diagnostic test: B. What are the results and will they help me in caring for my patients? *JAMA* 1994;**271**:703–7

3   Schon D. *The Reflective Practitioner: How Professionals Think in Action*. New York: Basic Books, 1983

4   Hansen MT, Nohria N, Tierney T. What's your strategy for managing knowledge? *Harvard Bus Rev* 1999;**77**:106–16, 187

5   Moran N. Knowledge is the key, whatever your sector. In: *Knowledge Management Survey*, Financial Times Business Solution Series. London: FT, 1999

6   Peckham M. Developing the National Health Service: a model for public services. *Lancet* 1999;**354**:1539–45

7   Ellis J, Mulligan I, Rowe J, Sackett D. Inpatient medicine is evidence based. *Lancet* 1995;**346**:407–10

8   Donaldson L. *An Organisation with Memory: Report of an Expert Group on Learning from Adverse Events in the NHS*. London: Stationery Office, 2000

9   Einbinder JS, Klein DA, Safran CS. Making effective referrals: a knowledge-management approach. *Proc AMIA Annu Fall Symp* 1997:330–4

10 O'Brien C, Cambouropoulos P. Combating information overload: a six-month pilot evaluation of a knowledge management system in general practice. *Br J Gen Pract* 2000;**50**:489–90

11 Go AS, Rao RK, Dauterman KW, Massie BM. A systematic review of the effects of physician specialty on the treatment of coronary disease and heart failure in the United States. *Am J Med* 2000;**108**:216–26

12 Bucknall CE, Robertson C, Moran F, Stevenson RD. Differences in hospital asthma management. *Lancet* 1988;**i**:748–50

13   Jadad AR, Haynes RB, Hunt D, Browman GP. The Internet and evidence-based decision-making: a needed synergy for efficient knowledge management in health care. *Can Med Assoc J* 2000;**162**:362–5

14   Matheson NW. Things to come: post-modern digital knowledge management and medical informatics. *J Am Med Inform Assoc* 1995;**2**:73–8

15   Gordon D, Hamscher W, King D, Mueller A, Parker B, Retter T, eds. Knowledge management. In: *Technology Forecast*. Menlo Park, CA: Price Waterhouse Coopers Technology Center, 2000:685–718

16   Jackson JR. The urgent call for knowledge management in medicine. *Physician Exec* 2000;**26**:28–31

17   Gray JM. Where's the chief knowledge officer? *BMJ* 1998;**317**:832

18   Vimarlund V, Timpka T, Patel VL. Information technology and knowledge exchange in health-care organisations. *Proc AMIA Annu Fall Symp* 1999:632–6

Index

NOTE: this index is in alphabetical order word by word. Page numbers in italic refer to tables